BUILD A NEW BODY

Build a New Body

Anthony Greenbank

NEW ENGLISH LIBRARY
TIMES MIRROR

First Published 1969 by Wolfe Publishing Ltd.
under the title of MISTER TOUGH

•

FIRST NEL PAPERBACK EDITION APRIL 1973

•

NEL Books are published by
New English Library Limited from Barnard's Inn, Holborn, London E.C.1.
Made and printed in Great Britain by Hunt Barnard Printing Ltd., Aylesbury, Bucks.

45001376 6

CONTENTS

INTRODUCTION

YOU can become MR TOUGH. Young or old, skinny or flabby, this book will unchain the Hercules hidden inside you—the Goliath lurking in every man who is medically sound yet way out of condition.

You—despite 20th century living destined to strip masculinity—ARE tough. Men in a crisis can wreak the violence of King Kong—yet be pimply/bald/bespectacled overweight or under-nourished figures.

Newspaper headlines prove this daily. . . . *Man lifts car off crash victim with bare hands; youth raced 70 m.p.h. express in level crossing drama; convict leaps 12 foot wall; buried-alive grave-digger claws way free; Chelsea pensioner fights off bank raiders; crane driver stops runaway cable—with teeth; father dives into river weir to save 2 sons.*

No fictional supermen these. But men in all kinds of fettle, far from being 100 per cent fit. Fear triggered their hidden reserves of nerve/brain/muscle to create a short-term Samson for them to use at will. Panic over, not one of them knew how they had done it.

How can YOU harness the toughness-craving release? What can YOU use as the trigger to grow muscles of whipcord/steel/titanium? Thanks to this book you no longer have to be afraid to become MR TOUGH.

Just eager to hot-up your body—the frame which has proved so resilient that ordinary men have been shot through the heart/had an iron bar through the head/been run over by a steamroller/swallowed by a whale/had 6,600 volt electric shock/been roasted in heat hot enough to cook steak . . . and lived.

STRENGTH is the norm of manhood—whether you are soon shattered love-making or pushing a stuck car, when it's paunches-in-quick as supergirl approaches or when running for a bus makes your lungs howl. Every man longs to keep his virility/vim/vigour.

Many strength books fail. Their theory of physiology, tables of calisthenics, training schedules put off most men who see themselves in a mad PT race—stopwatch in one fist, tape-measure in the other.

MR TOUGH is not like that. There are no timetables/schedules/treatises. YOU are as tough as you secretly feel and if—like millions—you *know* you are MR SOFT but hanker to change things, then here's how. Here is how to be as strong as you want, as tough as you *want* to feel. All you need is a body in medically sound condition. And burning determination to start now.

MR TOUGH says here is an arm. Here is how to rip a telephone directory in half *now* (without cheating or exercising a muscle). Here is how to work on that limb for a fortnight to reveal growing muscles. And here is how to build on those 14-days with a choice of exercises to convert that arm into a thudding piston with a *real* big end (YOU).

There is no secret route to strength—no *one* way. MR TOUGH, however, masses all power-triggers from peak-hour (everyone has one some time of day) exercising to yoga, from Strongman Stunts to Iron Game weight training. Cross references link body zones: each exercise attacks *different* slabs of muscle meaning a bonus every time you exercise.

Which MR TOUGH is YOU? Power-champion who blows up hot water bottles like balloons/bends 6 in. nails in fists/rips card decks in half? Or the A1 model (slim/fit/agile at *any* age). Pick the strengths you *want* from a tremendous choice. Win them using methods graded easy/hard: it depends on your present condition which you use.

But a Samson/Hercules/Goliath! Too much to believe? NO! Legends lie between what the average male to-day IS and CAN become. A man at 70 can better his physique 50 per cent; at 16 or 50, 75 per cent; at 30, 100 per cent. Men between 27 and 50 are often 8 years ahead of their age in bodily decay (motorists are 10).

MR TOUGH is **not** a WORLD'S FIRST EFFORTLESS EXERCISER. It takes grit/graft/guts to build physique whether only for a more manly torso or for a body like an ox. Even isometrics (armchair muscle-making) hurt when done with zip. But MR TOUGH will *bore* you through the effort-barrier in gripping style—never boring *you.*

Try using MR TOUGH this way: (1) read Chapter 1—a self-contained booklet on fitness in itself—and carry out its advice as you read, (2) read the rest, (3) re-read Chapter 1; plan a power programme *really* to toughen you (4) keep re-reading Chapter 1 throughout training.

See yourself now as MR TOUGH (we left his face blank so yours will fit). Skip worries that, because of your nature, you may always be pallid/small/shortsighted. Or well on in years. Your Goliath is waiting to explode. MR TOUGH can do YOU nothing but a power of good.

BODY

BODY: 1

YOUR BODY is a fortress. Its army of 700 muscles—half *your* mass—are "muscled" by 250 million fibres. Around each fibre are blood vessels so tiny that 400 will cram into a piece of muscle as skinny as a drawbridge splinter.

Battlements of bone can stand cruel seiges (a shin bone will jack up two tons; a skull can be crushed to within 10 per cent of its breadth before cracking). Ligament chains from bones to organs will lug 1,000 lb. weights.

Yet are YOU a ruin? A chest as bony as a portcullis or a gut as soft as hot lead mean a shorter/poorer/weaker life. Muscle-up with MR TOUGH and YOU can trample the ramparts of fitness and strength: KING of YOUR CASTLE.

WHAT MUSCLES CAN DO

Muscle minus fibrous supporting and packing tissue = the consistency of badly set jelly desert. Just look what men have done with it. . . .

Lifted 3-ton elephant one-handed. Torn 3 packs of cards in one go. Cracked a Brazil nut between shoulder blades. Smashed wine bottle gripped in crook of arm by swelling bicep. Shoved 40-ton truck up incline on rails. Bent bars of iron cage to escape. Blown bottom out of a milk bottle in one puff. Ripped pennies with teeth. Bent half-crowns with fingers. Lifted ¼-ton with one finger. Snapped barbed wire wrapped tight round bare chest with one gasp. Pulled a team of carthorses to standstill solo-handed. Fisted a hole through a brick wall.

HOW YOU CAN BE STRONGER INSTANTLY

Develop power in 300 muscles NOW. Boost them whether fat/fifty/forlorn. You need three things:

Strong motive. Want/want/want strength enough to murder unfit body for a new carcase because you stand to gain . . .

Respect. Self-respect. Self-confidence. Admiration. Friends. Girl friends. Sinews to burst wristwatch strap clasp/muscles to make shirts strangle you/fists to burst driving gloves. A flat belly. V-shaped torso. He-man's voice. Staying power. Endurance. Virility. Vice-style hand shake. Cat-lazy movement. Clearer/faster/potent thinking. Slow-throbbing pulse. Clearway circulation. Boyhood vim. Suppleness. Least chance of heart attack/backache/asthma. Deep sleep. Nerve. Bouncing energy. Giant spirit. Better hanger for suits. Survival.

Pinpoint concentration. Aim eyeballs. Grit teeth. Narrow eyes. Plant feet. Square shoulders. Aim eyeballs. Flex toes. Grunt/growl/groan. Grasp bar. Aim eyeballs. Stamp feet. Row oars. Catch sandbag. S-t-r-e-t-c-h. Aim eyeballs. Pump arms. Gasp breath. Spread toes. Tighten grip. Whiten knuckles. Lash out. Aim eyeballs. Brain punchbag. Skip rope. Push/pull/push. Shove harder. Gasp in. Tilt jaw. Shrug shoulders. Aim eyeballs. Aim eyeballs. Aim eyeballs.

Note: concentrate intensely seeing nothing in front of you—eyeballs focussed on only one target: boosting muscles to utmost potential you desire.

Lack of inhibition. Don't stop to think about it—do it. In private. Solo. Alone. Cut-off. In secret. Keep away from others until proud of physique. Nothing else exists. Go-Go-Go. Give it stick. Move it/move it/move it. Fight it/fight it/fight it. Bomb your body. Blitz those muscles. Try/try/try. Unwind. Forget failures. Let go. GO-GO-GO. Pile it on. Ram it home. Skip age-complex. Think young. Train young. Look young.

UNLEASH TIGER POWER NOW

Confirm 3-secrets of power to-day with strength feats. *Motive* = to astonish friends. *Concentration* makes feats possible for most men. So does *lack of inhibition* (you tried them first alone, discovered knack).

Remember: do feats in proportion to present strength (lift light tables etc. now, heavy ones later). Put up a struggle as you concentrate. Finish off feats with big flourish. Never confide secret of your power to anyone.

Dent a beer can with your finger

Take FULL pint-sized beer can (or soup/bean/milk tin). And grip it onehanded (with welded metal seam against hand palm). Diag. 1

1. PLACE FOREFINGER ON TABLE* AS SHOWN
2. PRESSDOWN HARD WITH MIDDLE JOINT.
3. HOLD CAN ABOVE FINGER AND . . .

4. BRING IT DOWN HARD TO HIT FINGER WITH CENTRE OF SIDE OF CAN.

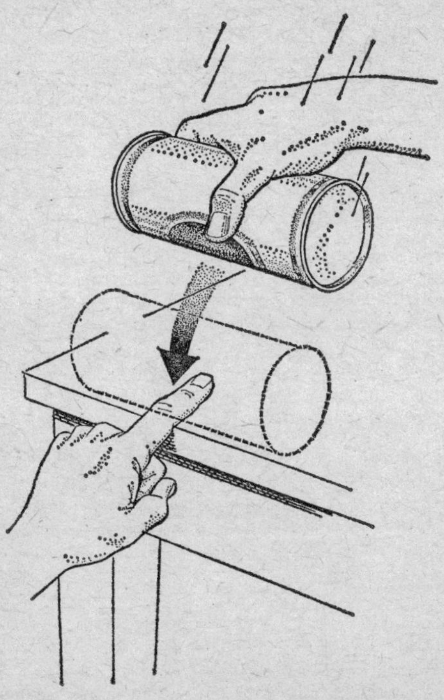

5. CAN IS DENTED, YOUR FINGER UNHURT.

Reason: YOUR finger is much tougher than you thought.

*= *take great care. Use large cans (more surface area to bend). Place ALL finger firmly on table OVER a table leg or some other structural support. Try bashing beer can across a pencil at first to practise blow/aim/idea. NEVER hit with can bottom/top edges.*

Now drink the beer (careful—it spurts out)—and if can is 1-pint size (or if you have dented a can of fruit juice/Coke/ lemonade about similar size) . . .

Tear the tin can in half with bare fists (at first: slowly/ cannilly/safely).

1. BASH IN DENT ALREADY MADE IN NOW EMPTY

CAN BY KARATE BLOW WITH EDGE OF HAND (EASY).

2. PRESS THUMBS ON DENT AND SQUEEZE CAN DOUBLE WITH BOTH FISTS.
3. GRIP ENDS OF CAN TWO-FISTED TO BEND IT OTHER WAY.
4. KEEP BENDING BACK/FORTH/BACK UNTIL . . .
5. CAN CAN BE TORN IN HALF TWO-FISTED ACROSS CENTRAL TEAR-LINE.

Keep practising on *empty* soup/beans/veg cans until YOU can rip a can bisectually in two grunts. Note: the longer the can the easier it is.

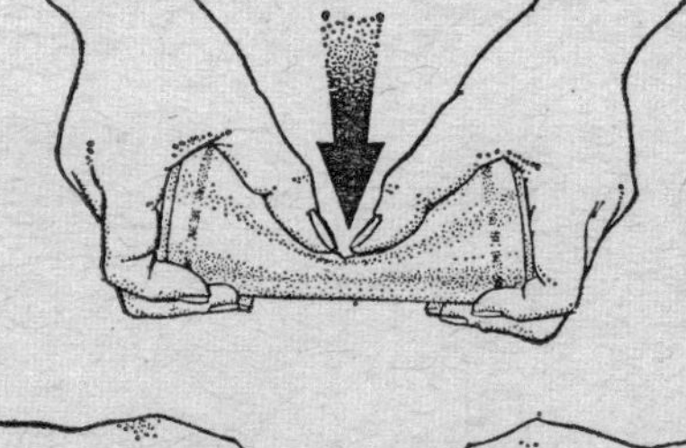

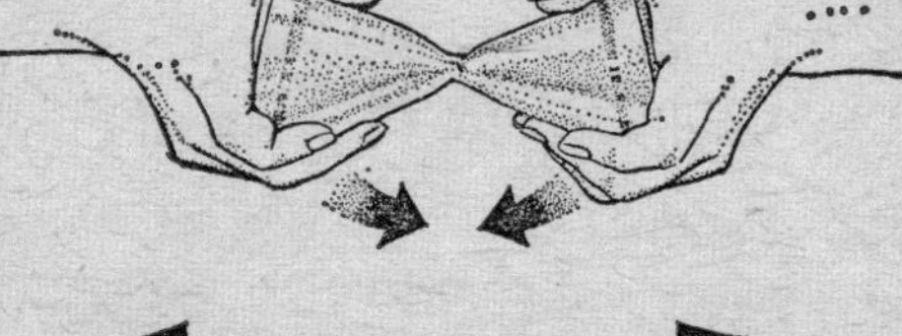

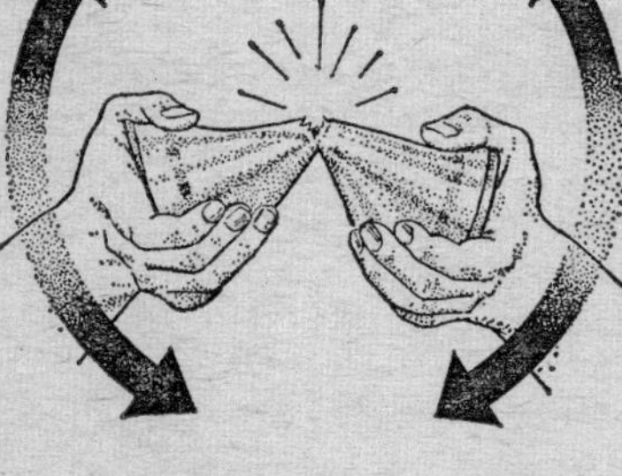

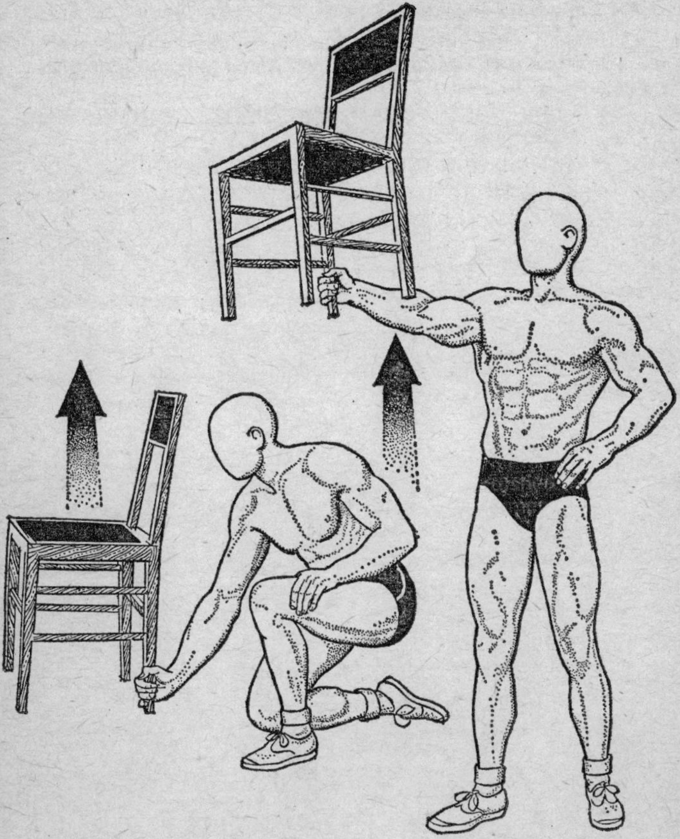

Snatch up a chair one-fisted by one leg

Practice with wooden kitchen chair. Bigger chairs later.

1. GO DOWN ON ONE KNEE BY CHAIR.
2. GRASP BOTTOM OF ONE LEG.
3. TIP CHAIR SLIGHTLY TOWARDS YOU WITH WRIST PULL.
4. LIFT CHAIR ABOVE HEAD OLYMPIC TORCH STYLE.

Easiest way = with bent elbow. Hardest way = straight-armed.

Rip a telephone directory in half

No previous baking in oven/tearing and regluing/other cheating. Practice first with wad of magazines. Then an old London A–D directory.

1. CURL FISTS ROUND PAGE EDGES (THUMBS ON TOP).
2. BEND BOOK UP/DOWN TO SOFTEN FIBRES.
3. SHIFT GRIP TO FEATHER-OUT PAGES.
4. ATTACK THINNEST PART OF ANGLED PAGES.
5. YANK UP AND OUT WITH STRONGEST HAND: DOWN WITH OTHER.
6. LOCK THUMBS IN PLACE.
7. REALLY RIP ONCE FEATHERING TEARS THROUGH.

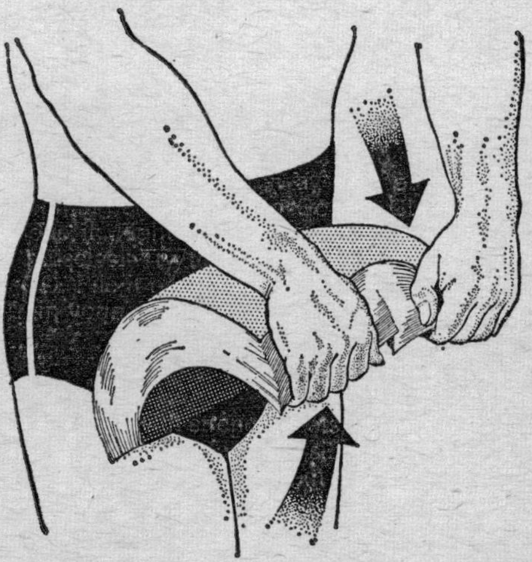

First half of feat is done slowly—second, violently as both fists seize thick wadges of paper.

Lift a man on a shovel

10–12 stones will do at first. Work up to 16-stone men.

1. STAND MAN SIDEWAYS ON SHOVEL (AS SHOWN).
2. BEND TO GRIP BASE AND END OF HANDLE.
3. TAKE STRONG GRASP, PROPPING LOWER ELBOW ON KNEE-INSIDE.

4. SAY: "I am definitely going to lift you high off the ground. Put your hands on my back so you can steady yourself as you go up."
5. JERK DOWN SHARPLY ON HANDLE END (SO MAN PRESSES ON BACK).
6. LIFT SHOVEL WITH ALL YOUR MIGHT.

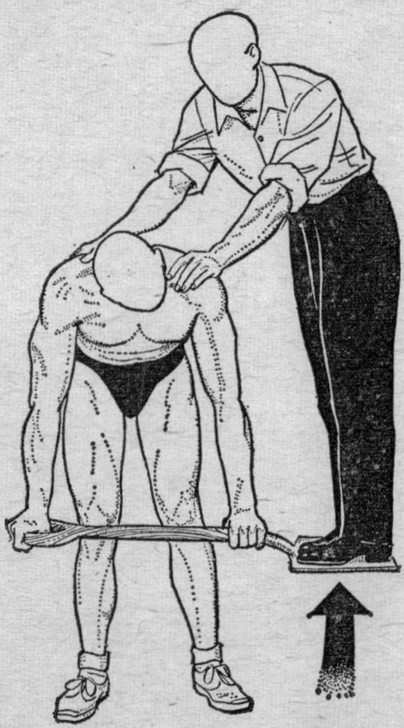

Timing/leverage/lift *will* raise man. First ¼ in. worst—rest is easy. Try on grass first. Hit method right first time and man can fly over your shoulder.

Carry 14 pints of beer

Or, if short-fingered, 12. With stubby fingers or weak left (or right) hand use this formula:

0 pints on little finger.
2 pints on 3rd finger.
1 pint on 2nd finger.
3 pints on forefinger + thumb.

With long fingers try for 14 pints this way.

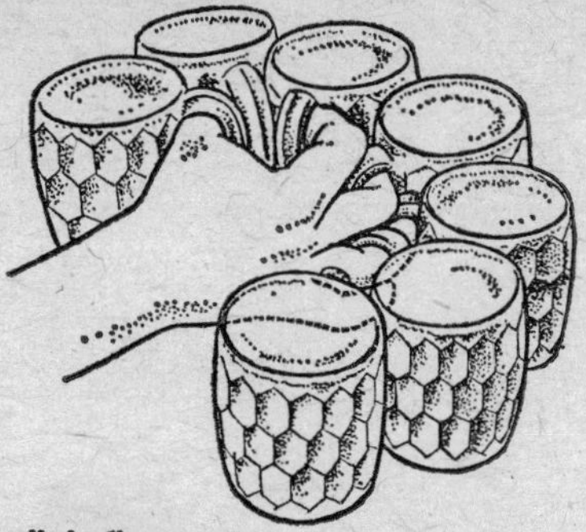

1 pint on little finger.
2 pints on 3rd finger.
1 pint on 2nd finger.
3 pints on forefinger + thumb.

Crystal ring of glass sides lever against each other to help you. Extra clearance rim of new mugs prevents slopping.

Outpull 4 men

Try with 2 men first, then with 4 as your strength booms.

1. STAND STRAIGHT/LEGS APART/FEET PLANTED FIRMLY.
2. RAISE ELBOWS AND CLASP HANDS IN FRONT OF CHEST.

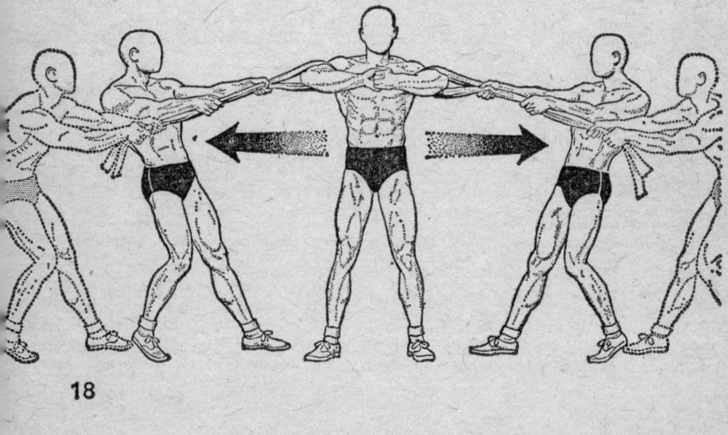

3. ENSURE FOREARMS CROSS NIPPLE LEVEL.
4. HAVE 2 MEN HOLD A TOWEL OVER EACH ELBOW.
5. TELL THEM TO PULL STEADILY TUG O' WAR STYLE.
6. YOUR CHAIN WILL HOLD.

Arms in this position = powerfully placed for any pull. Also—pullers get poor traction.

YOUR HERCULES REVEALED

THIS Giant exists in all men (YOUR forearm muscles can hoist own 12 oz.* weight 100 feet in one spasm *now*). Only surface muscle shown—more lies in internal organs.

* *12 oz. = weight of 48 pennies.*

Muscles

1. STERNOMASTOID steers head with twin reins of muscle roping breastbone top to rear of ears.
2. DELTS (*Deltoids*) piston arms with cylinder head muscle topping arms/shoulders.
3. PECS (*Pectorals*) bellow chest and bullock arms (in/back/down) with breastplate muscles.
4. BICEPS jacknife lower arm to upper limb with muscle bulge fronting upperarm.
5. VASTUS INTERNUS snaps out leg/steadies knee joint with inside thigh muscle (can correct crooked thighs).
6. TIBS (*Tibialis Anticus*) kicks foot up towards knee with shinpad muscle.
7. RECTUS FEMORIS straightens leg/flexes knee joint with thighshield muscle.
8. SARTORIOUS flexes hip/knee joints and sidekicks leg with flat strap of muscle buckling hip to knee.
9. EXTERNAL OBLIQUES turn trunk/swivel spine with corset of slanting muscle.
10. ABS (*Abdominals*) flexes trunk on pelvis and empties chest with corrugated muscle wall.
11. SERRATUS MAGNUS balloons chest and floats shoulder blades with rafts of chestside muscle.
12. TRAPS (*Trapezius*) fly shoulders (and blades) with big flat kite of muscle on back of neck.
13. LATS (*Latissimus Dorsi*) rows arms/twists trunk/boosts breathing with muscle fanning from waist to armpits.
14. FLEXORS AND EXTENSORS control hand palm with 20 sinewy muscles through wrist.
15. GLUTES (*Gluteals*) cushion thighs with backside muscle complex.

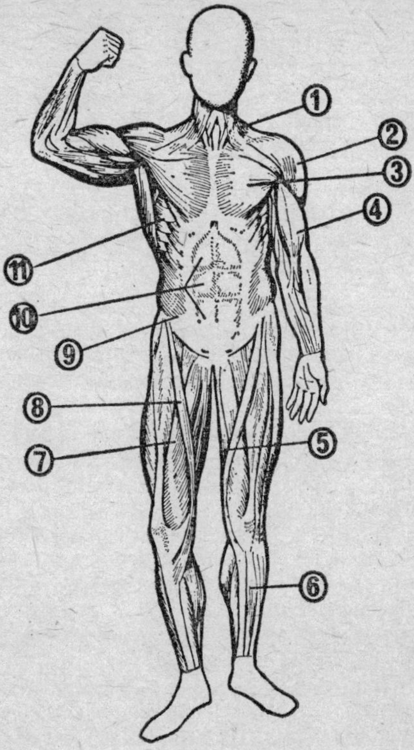

16. GASTROS (*Gastrocnemius*) lifts heel/points toes out/ flexes knee with calf muscle mound.
ERECTOR SPINAE cranes body upright with 2 spine-side tow ropes of muscle. (*Not shown.*)

17. ACHILLES TENDON hauls heel with muscular yank of 500 lbs. a step making it toughest tendon.

18. HAMSTRINGS penknife lower legs to thigh with back thigh biceps-style muscle group.

19. TRICEPS fist out arms and can (+biceps+brachialis) freeze arm rigid with rearguard upper arm muscle.

20. BRACHIALIS folds-up lower arm (like biceps) with frontview muscle on upper arm.

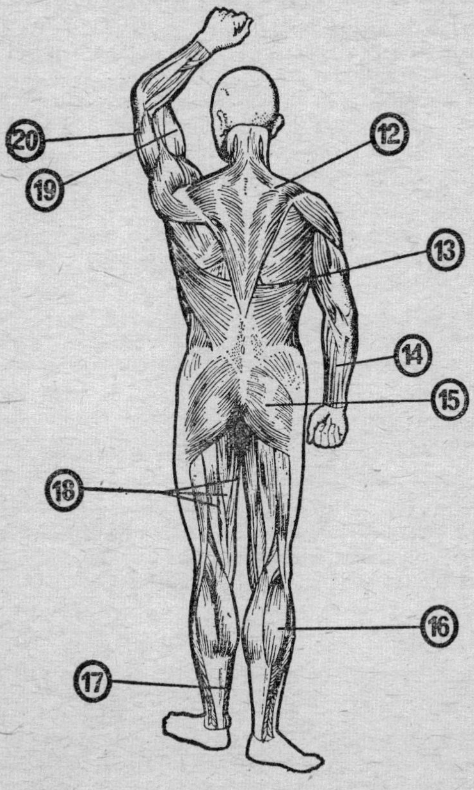

Also going for you . . .

MILLIONS of living cells (less than 1/100th inch long).

5 QUARTS of blood to sluice away exercise-wrecked muscle debris—and to flood new-growing muscle with oxygen/food.

HEART (YOUR toughest muscle) beats 38 million times yearly, pumps 4,320 gallons of blood a day, expends energy equivalent to hoisting a ton 82 feet.

750 MILLION air sacs in lungs working 21,600 times a day.

GASTRIC JUICES able to dissolve metal but not stomach walls.

LIVER which CAN turn body fat into glucose.

2 KIDNEYS as big as fists each storing 1,000,000 filters for blood—to purify 200 quarts of blood a day.

206 BONES hinged by self-oiling joints, bound by ligament.

NERVOUS SYSTEM via spinal column and beyond where impulses travel at 300 m.p.h.

SKIN acting as a second lung (pulls in oxygen, pushes out waste); as a sun blotter (traps Vitamin D); as a body barometer (boils/spots/dryness can = hidden tension).

TENDONS of white cord tissue binding muscle to bone.

JOINTS (ball & socket/hinge/gliding).

GLANDS powering nerve/mental/muscle boost when body is threatened by upkicking hormone production via pituitary, stomach, thymus, adrenal glands . . . and undamming torrent of strength.

NOURISH YOUR HIDDEN GIANT NOW

Pasty-faced/scrawny necked/bow legged a man can gain health and strength (and better looks) within days. Tone-up the Titan-within to-day.

Supercharge circulation

S-T-R-E-T-C-H-I-N-G = blood transfusion *into* muscles. Reach out a lot. Like a cat. Slowly. Best when a habit (NOT just tired when body stretches automatically). Other good ways: rotate shoulder girdle; contract and relax spine; stretch-and-shorten neck.

Electrify skin

Have bath/shower/rough-cloth-chest-rinse *every* day. Always chill down with cool *not* cold water. Skip scalding baths. Frosty baths OK if you say. Cool off warm bath with fast tap jet. Rub down roughly with brisk towel. Use good deodorant but never anti-perspirant (sweat is natural). NEVER use hot water/soap/rubbing on face (especially if rotten complexion). Instead (1) use tepid water face wash (2) finger-on hair shampoo lather (3) rinse with lukewarm water (4) swill with aftershave or waterfall-cold water (5) blot face dry with paper towels. Feed bad complexions with baby lotion overnight.

Bombard skin (in direct contact with nervous system) with sun/rain/wind. Never overdo sunbathing if whiteskin: short bursts best until tanned. Buy *good* sunray lamp. Rain running/dew rolling/snow surfing = great. Fresh air to skin = golden hide hiding robe of muscle.

Tone-up teeth

Tourniquet any Dracula-look with dental surgery (worth cash to

YOUR confidence). Table salt excellent tooth whitener/gum healer/teeth tightner. If you lose salt/toothpaste try soot (excellent). Brush twice daily. Yellow molars = X-film Horror (rid film with very occasional powdered pumice stone brushings). Chew gum/gargle lemon juice/salt-brush for freshest breath.

Highlight hair

Wash when dirty. Use Stergene. Saliva = best hair fixer. Also water (*brush* watered hair until stray hairs lie with others); *comb* still-damp hair into shape; comb-flick dry hair later. Stays set for hours. Pay more for better haircuts.

Cut down clothing

Do it gradually (like paratroopers condition for cold). Don't wear too many (many do). Discard cardigans/Long Johns/etc. slowly. One by one. Overclothing = less fight to colds/chills/bugs. Makes you too hot unknowingly—cuts down body efficiency.

Buy fewer clothes. But best quality affordable. Same with shoes. Change underwear/socks/shirts each day. Keep suits pressed, often dry cleaned. Care for shoes like you do for feet.

Check with doctor . . .

. . . if in ANY doubt ANYTIME about health. Have confirmation *THAT* . . . ghostly face = blood vessels further under skin than usual NOT anaemia nor being off-colour; *THAT* sudden chest pains = dyspepsia (thro' big meals before bed) NOT heart attack; *THAT* from 15–45 you CAN gain strength/endurance; *THAT* from 45 you WILL win fitness/teenage vim; *THAT* exercising DOES heart good (a muscle like biceps); *THAT* exercise after illness IS good; *THAT* 80-year-olds CAN keep a flat gut and fit.

Note: men in 40s must not act tougher than they are. BUT they can build-up power gradually until they ARE tough-enough for hard exercise.

Be a calorie miser*

(**= energy value of food measured in heat units.*)

Don't squander calories by burning up energy wastefully. Rest during day in hour periods. Do nothing. Sit, feet up. Doze. Lazybone it. Take a sauna bath. Have your back stroked (usually free). Rest after sex (good sex is good for you). Read. Listen to music you love. Smoke cigarette (just one). Sip beer. Unwind mind. Loosen up. Daydream. Curl up. Slacken sinews. Save calories needed for muscle tissue.

Relax 30 minutes before each meal. Avoid arguments/excitement/animation while eating. Switch off TV during meal. Eat slowly, quietly (if excited/upset food is not digested properly for muscle-making). Take slow 15 minute walk afterwards OR skip activity for 60 minutes.

Grow muscles in sleep

Sleep well. Like a log. Buy a *good* bed. Read yourself to sleep. Play radio. Take warm drink. Encourage sleep. Aim for 9 hours in bed a night. Muscles grow in sleep (scientific fact). You save calories (used-up by lack of sleep). Improve nerves (ruined by insomnia). Body-feel = best barometer whether you slept well. Note: try deep breathing to fall asleep. Or exercise first. Check bedroom well-ventilated/bladder drained/curtains drawn (to cut out dawn). Throw away pyjamas (naked sleepers sleep best).

And if too cold—use hot water bottle. BUT *not* for feet. Hug it. Or good woman (sex = BEST sleepmaker).

Dose-up with oxygen

Pep yourself up ANYTIME. Tank up with oxygen. Make it a habit (NOT just when yawning = Nature's way of boosting oxygen intake to wake you up when tired).

Do 10-minute breathing spells when walking thus: inhale hard for 4 steps, hold breath another 4 (count as you step out), exhale slowly over 5 steps.

Breathe easily/evenly/deeply.

If above formula out of step with YOU try: inhale for 3 steps, exhale for 5. Or inhale for 5 steps, exhale for 8. Choose best method for you.

When doing first time, practise in garden rather than High Street, where there's a lot of traffic—(over-oxygenation can lead to dizziness); extremely difficult to keep up your breathing schedule if pinned under front wheel of bus.

Another oxygen booster: roll head three times slowly in each direction. Gasp in deep breaths. Blow-out in sharp bursts through gritted teeth and pursed lips. It works for short periods.

Don't wreck yourself

Smoking/drinking/lovemaking all right unless you smoke like a chimney/drink like a fish/etc. (up to 15 cigarettes a day OK). Watch who you kiss/touch/contact. Syphillis/hepatitis/athlete's foot will KO any budding Hercules. Keep clean habits (no drinking from others' beer, etc.). Avoid dirty people, germ-ridden areas. Keep off aphrodisiacs/happiness/love pills (Spanish Fly burns guts and kills). Opium/hash/cocaine conjure erotica, NOT virility. Sleeping tablets and slimming drugs are out.

Devour a NEW body

You ARE what you eat.

Muscles store vital power you get from food. Never eat just to satisfy appetite—work out right food to grow muscle tissue. Note: eating too much/wrong foods = you go fat with a calorie surplus. Less chance of dying from 15 cigarettes a day than from being 10 lbs. overweight (every extra 1 lb. of fat = $\frac{1}{4}$ mile of blood vessels).

Mix food into *balanced* diet.

1. EAT SMALLER MEALS MORE OFTEN.

2. DRINK AT LEAST 3 PINTS LIQUID DAILY.

3. MISS WRONG FOODS SUCH AS WHITE BREAD, POTATOES, SWEETS, REFINED SUGAR, PASTRIES, CANNED GOODS, FROZEN FOODS.

4. EAT UNREFINED NOSH SUCH AS HARD RYE BREAD (OR WHOLE WHEAT GRAIN), UNREFINED SUGAR, RAW SALADS, GREENEST VEGETABLES, NUTS, CHEESE, MILK, UNPOLISHED RICE, FRUIT.

5. SCOFF PILES OF PROTEIN (GOLDEN NUGGETS OF NUTRITION WHICH FEED MUSCLE): LEAN MEAT, CURDS, CHEESE, EGGS, MILK, FISH.

6. AVOID TOO MANY CARBOHYDRATES (SUGAR/BREAD/POTATOES) AND FATS WHICH POUR OUT ENERGY BUT FATTEN YOU IF GOBBLED GANNET-STYLE.

7. TO SLIM: GOOD DIET SATISFIES HUNGER. CUT DOWN SUGAR/STARCH (BUT DON'T CUT DOWN *ALL* CARBOHYDRATES/FATS). EAT LESS. LET BODY FEED ON RESERVES. HAVE BIG NOSH NOW AND THEN. DON'T STARVE. RELY MAINLY ON PROTEINS (DRINK MILK-SHAKE-TYPE PROTEIN SUPPLEMENTS* SHOWN IN MUSCLE MAG ADS). EAT NOTHING BETWEEN MEALS. CUT DOWN ON LIQUIDS.
   **= good at any time.*

8. TO ADD BULK: EAT MORE GOOD FOOD. BACON FAT, BUTTER, CHEESE, MILK, CREAM, DATES, EGGS, NUTS, FIGS, HONEY, MARGARINE, OLIVE OIL, RAISINS, RICE, SUGAR, HALIBUT, POTATOES, BREAD, AND DRINK PINTS.

9. EAT MINERALS: CALCIUM FROM CHEESE/RAISINS/OATMEAL; IODINE FROM FISH/IODIZED SALT/WATERCRESS; SODIUM FROM TABLE SALT.

10. SKIP FRIED FOODS.

11. FOODS BEST EATEN RAW. DON'T OVERCOOK MEAT. POTATOES BEST IN JACKETS (EAT THESE TOO). USE GREENS WATER IN SOUPS/STEWS.

12. TO COMBAT ACNE/BLACKHEADS/GREASY SKIN: LEAVE ALONE BAKED BEANS, CANNED SALMON, PORK, POTATOES, PIES, PEANUT BUTTER, OILS, CANNED FRUIT, DRIED PEAS/BEANS, CHOCOLATE, BUTTER, BANANAS.

13. GET PLENTY OF VITAMINS.

These are . . .

Vitamin A attacks infection (*halibut, cod liver oil, animal fats, carrots, tomatoes, milk, greens*).

B bolsters nervous system/boosts appetite/buttresses fertility (*yeast, wheat germ, unpolished cereals, liver*).

B2 battles skin infections (*egg yolk, wholemeal flour, yeast, almonds, cheese, eggs*).

C creates bones/cradles teeth/cures muscle soreness (*raw greens, oranges, lemons, grapefruit, tomatoes*).

D doses bones and teeth (*halibut, cod liver oil, meat fat, eggs, butter, herrings, pork, liver, tuna, salmon, sun*).

E energises muscle/reproductive systems (*meats, eggs, leaves of greens, butter, carrots, celery, eggs, sprouts, spinach*).

KNOW YOUR STRENGTH TO-DAY

Try yourself. Use quick test as progress convincer/muscle fan club/milestick to toughness throughout your training.

Miss out easy exercises in book if you gain high scores.

Muscle Power

Face wall, feet together. Reach to limit with both arms and chalk-mark limit on wall. Now stand sideways. Bend knees. Swing arms. J-u-m-p. And reach with chalk one-handed. Mark wall at limit of jump reach. Measure gap between 2 marks.

Less $17\frac{1}{4}$ in.	= very poor muscle power.
$17\frac{1}{4}$ in.–$18\frac{1}{2}$ in.	= poor.
$18\frac{1}{2}$ in.–$19\frac{1}{2}$ in.	= fair.
$19\frac{1}{2}$ in.–$20\frac{1}{2}$ in.	= average.
$20\frac{1}{2}$ in.–$21\frac{1}{2}$ in.	= good.
$21\frac{1}{2}$ in.–23 in.	= very good.
Over 23 in.	= muscle power excellent.

Stomach muscle state

Lie flat. Arm straight, palms on thighs. Keep chin on chest. Sit up raising head, sliding hands down thighs till fingertips touch knees. Then reverse. Uncurl till flat on back. Repeat movement (counting) until body has had enough with legs flat on floor.

Minus 6	=	poor.
6–10	=	not good.
11–18	=	fair.
19–27	=	average.
28–37	=	good.
38–48	=	very good.
Over 49	=	excellent stomach muscles.

Stamina

Do step-ups on to wooden kitchen chair at 30 a minute rate for 5 minutes (150 up/down). Non-stop. Rest a minute. Count pulse* during next 30 secs. Wait 30 secs more then repeat 30-sec pulse count. Rest 90 secs. Take another 30-sec pulse count. Add 3 pulse counts together. Divide total into 15,000.

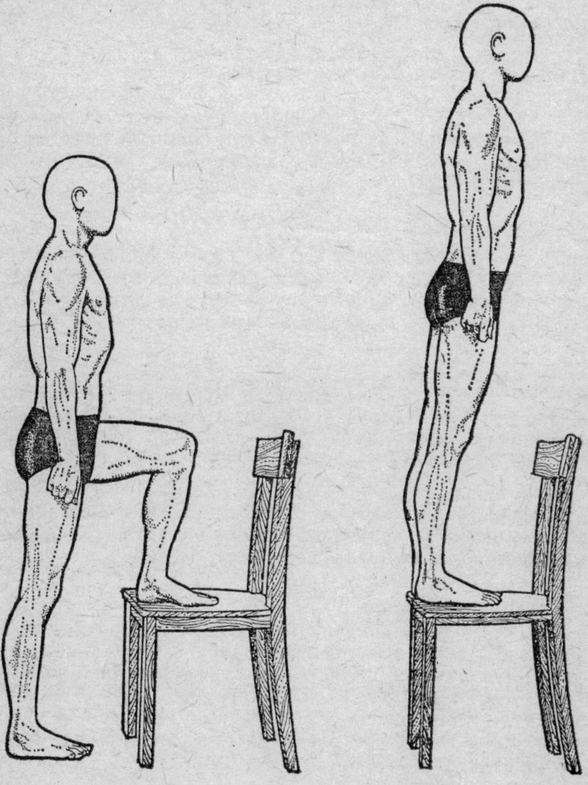

Minus 71	=	very poor.
71–74	=	poor.
75–80	=	fair.
81–87	=	average.
88–94	=	good.
95–110	=	very good.
Over 110	=	excellent stamina.

* Grip right wrist palm up in left hand. Curl left hand fingers and press tightly on right hand side of tendons just under horizontal wrinkles. Count number of beats a minute.

FITTER IN A FORTNIGHT

You can feel fighting fit in 14 days. With a glow that shows/amazes you/makes friends look. Fitter, remember—*strength* comes later.

Don't ruin yourself—run yourself in

Exercise in easy stages at first. Never aim for power pronto. Use common sense. Forget punishing exercises at first (lying on back, raising feet and legs high). Run body in slowly (astonishing what it can stand). Don't give sudden shocks to muscles—will strain joints/muscle/ligaments. Oil muscles (no toil).

Try cheating

Sensible when unfit. Clamp feet under bed if finding them airborne while raising body off floor. Or keep legs apart, knees bent a bit and touch toes with one hand not two. Or do press-ups from knees, not toes. As power returns cut out cheating.

Expect aches

Normal in few days after exercising starts. Shows you need working on. Don't despair if winded. Aches will go once you make habit of fitness.

Keep at it

NEVER give up. Use self discipline/hard graft/keenness. Know no lazy way. Keep to planned sessions each week. Don't get side-tracked. Next 14 days vital for YOU.

Don't expect miracles

Go for long-term improvement. Some progress happens in 2 weeks BUT only a start to end potential. Don't bet on big muscles in a few weeks. Shape is as individual as fingerprints—3 basic moulds exist: Michelin Man/Oxfam Ad/Boy Wonder. Start to get best of yours NOW. Quickest size gains = round chest/biceps. Possible to put 2 in. on expanded chest in 14 days with weights (progress takes longer after this).

Note: Boy Wonder physique has head start BUT *all* bodies can be improved immeasurably.

Don't shout about it
Let hardening body speak for you—not a big mouth. Keep quiet while growing fit/strong/tough. Don't shout the odds. Nor give scope for mickey-taking. Nor behave like a fresh air fanatic. Workout in private. Be purposeful/determined/laconic. And totally non-lunatic.

Workout properly
In well-ventilated room. Not hot/fuggy/smokey. Keep warm—away from draughts. Anywhere (shed/attic/bedroom) will do so long as can swing arms and lie on floor. Turn off gas while exercising. Wear bathing trunks/sweater. Or loose clothing minus buckles/straps round waist. Pumps or barefeet = OK.

NEVER workout with full stomach (pick time at least hour from meal, preferably 2 hours). Breathe through mouth in great gulps—IN on making effort. Exhale hard with hiss. AVOID toe-touching or sit-up exercises if overweight and paunchy (only do these when body slims and effort is not hell).

Afterwards—take alternate h. & c. shower/bath/chest rinse. Wrap up. Let body cool down slowly.

PLAN your fortnight
80 per cent potential MR TOUGHS drop out. Don't burn off MR SOFT by: trying to hustle muscle; punishing/torturing/scourging body; over-doing it; exhausting body on elaborate programme.

Farm body on simple plan for 14 days.

1. PLOUGH EXERCISE INTO EACH NIGHT.

2. PITCHFORK INTO FOLLOWING WORKOUT ROUTINE FOR 14 DAYS.

3. DON'T THRESH MORE THAN 10 REPS* PER EXERCISE IN FIRST WEEK NOR 12 REPS THE SECOND WEEK.

   **reps = revs:* 1/2/3/4/5/6/*etc.*

4. IF IT TAKES TRACTORLOADS OF EFFORT TO REACH THESE REP FIGURES ADD ANOTHER WEEK OR TWO UNTIL EASIER.

5. COUNT THIS AS VITAL CONDITIONING PERIOD BEFORE ALL ELSE IF UNFIT.

Exercise
As follows . . .

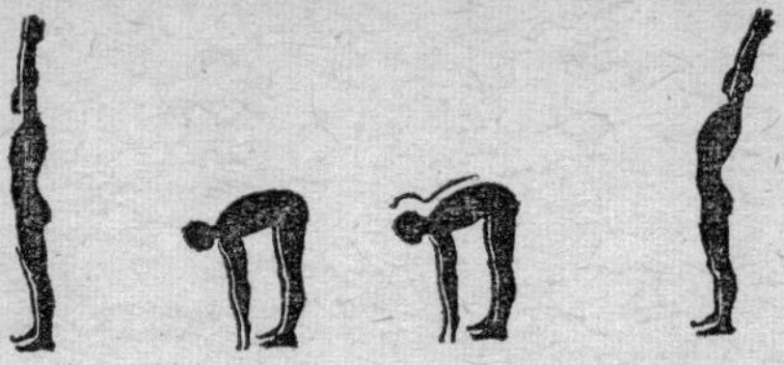

(a) Stand astride. Bend down to touch toes. Don't be depressed if you fail toe-contact at first.

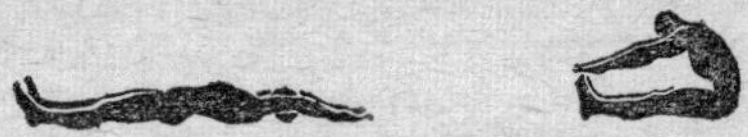

(b) Lie down. Stretch arms past head. Try to touch toes on sitting-up keeping knees flat down.

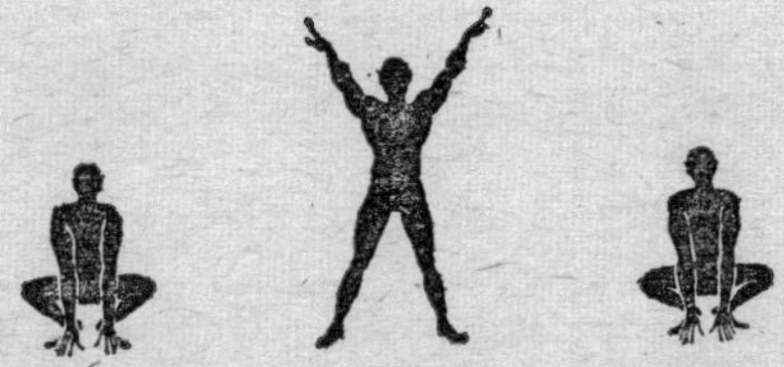

(c) Squat, crouched. Hands on floor. Spring up spanning arms and legs. Come down again in a crouch.

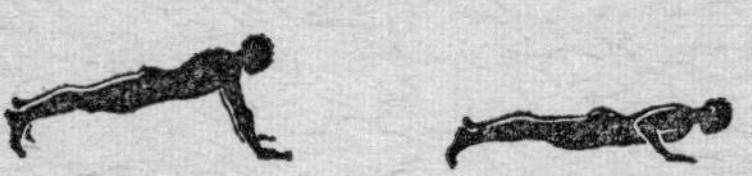

(d) Push-ups. Keep body as straight as possible. Aim not to touch floor as you go down.

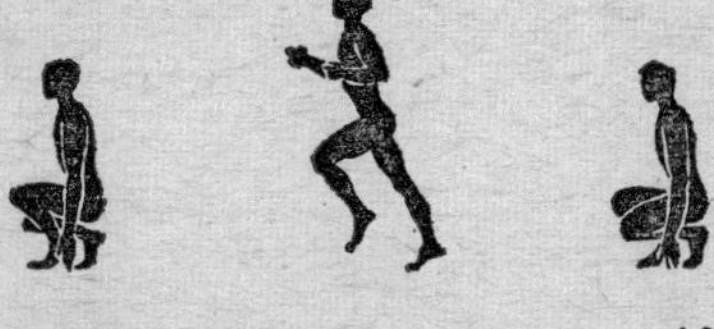

(e) Duck walk 5 steps, then run on spot 10 steps before going down again.

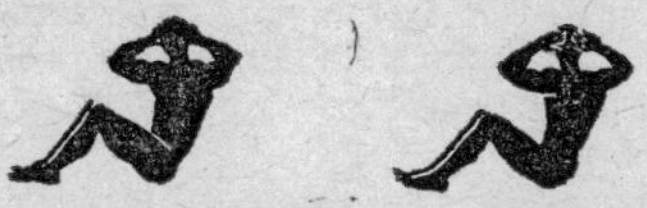

(f) Sit, knees bent. Hands behind head, Swivel body first one way, then the other, touching elbows to knees.

(g) Lie face down, hands clasped behind back. Lift head and legs off floor.

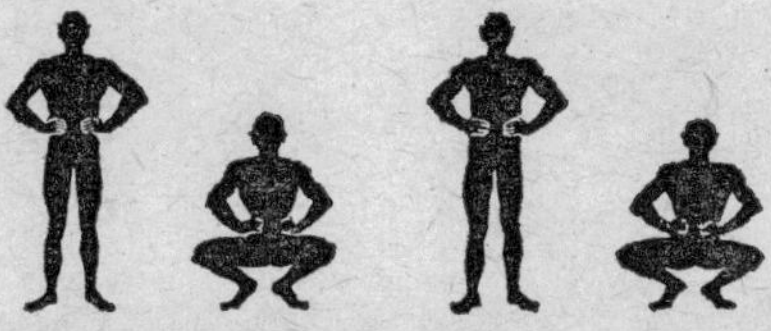

(h) Go down double knees bend, hands on hips (or held out front to keep balance). Straighten up.

OR

carry out mini-plan of four easy loosening-up workouts if very unfit/old/fat. Carry them out same way (there is NO one set of exercises, NO secret elixir, NO one system to toughen body (Manchester City do these).

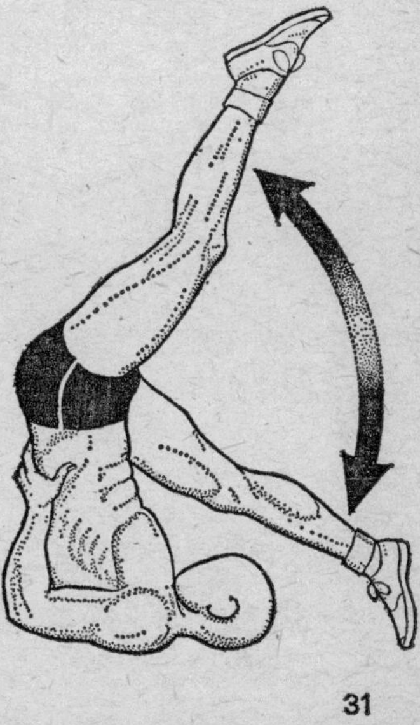

(i) Press back on floor with feet in air (hands on small of back). Alternately touch toes at back of head on floor.

(j) Stand legs apart and straight, arms stretched in same direction, swinging from left to right to work trunk.

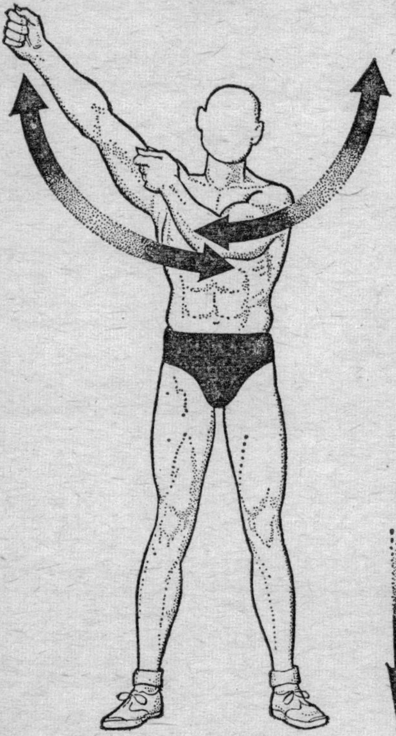

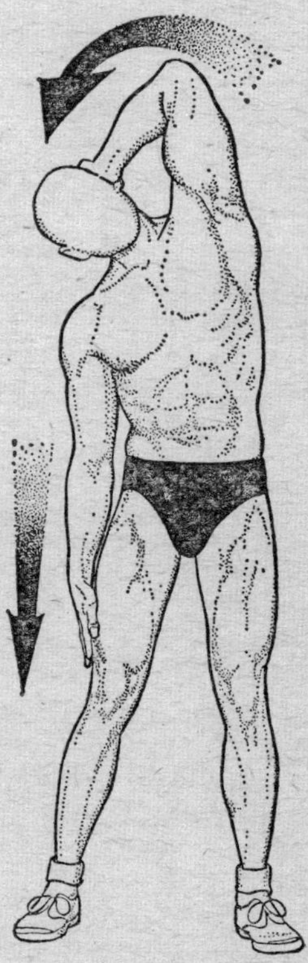

(k) Stand legs straight and apart, one hand on one side of head, other on leg. Push down and back as far as possible.

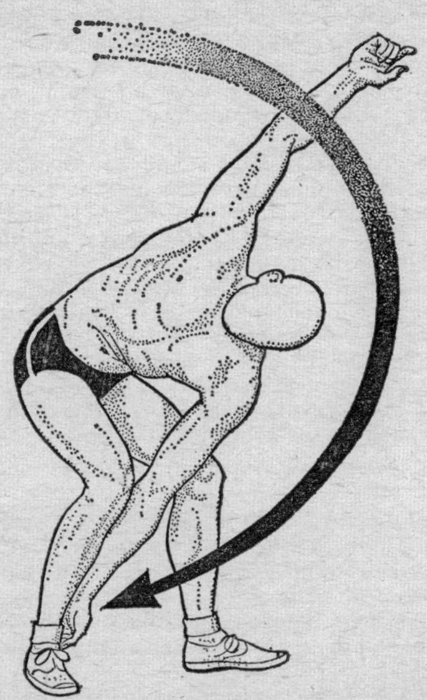

(l) Stand legs apart. Alternately touch back of left foot with right hand and vice versa swinging other hand for balance.

Remember: if you feel you are failing *do what you can*. Persevere until body allows full reps. Take first 2 weeks easily. Only go harder when body signals green: you *feel* pink condition. Take longer than 14 days if necessary.

MUSCULAR IN MONTHS

Biceps $1\frac{1}{4}$ in. extra in 2 months; $2\frac{1}{2}$ in. more in 5 months (tape measure not needed: shirt sleeve tension tells). You FEEL the difference all over.

Be as tough as you want

You can become so. Nothing can stop a determined YOU. YOU CAN do it. No barrier exists YOU cannot crash with runaway will.

One MR UNIVERSE had had both legs crushed and steel pins slotted in. World-beater muscle champ didn't start till 30. Olympic weight-lifter had spine surgery at 40—still hoists like a derrick. 45-year-old written off by doctors won 26-mile marathon at 54 against teen-and-twenties rivals. Tennis champ plays at 70 like 30 year old. 80-year-old scaled Matterhorn.

You CAN do it. Once fitness gained from "free" exercises (as done earlier), strength comes from progressive resistance to muscle (using body weight/body tension/low cost gear as THE resistance).

Give it everything. YOU are as tough as YOU feel: many feel soft now but, with enthusiastic workouts, can soon gain toughness-feel until body/soul/mind says STOP. Depends on age/outlook/condition when HALT flicks you off to individual fitness-level. It may be soon or never: you win either way.

Choose own MR TOUGH. Muscle Beach King.* Skinny canoe paddler Eskimo rolling in rapids. Fit/wiry/tanned executive in irridescent suit. Droopy 6-footer scaling Exit Cracks on North Wall of Eiger. Survivor in car crash/building fall/office fire. Caveman Conquistador at parties. Old age pensioner with flat stomach and zest. Tawny male model with grip of chrome molybdenum. Schoolboy Nobby Stiles.

* *Not all girlybirds go for Muscle Beach Monarchs whatever muscle ads say.*

NEVER feel worst physical wreck in town. Use self-criticism as spur not saddle. THINK way to strength/power/stamina. Forget age. Again, **thinking** young = **looking** young.

Age/hereditary/rib-cage-size ALL determine physical potential (some's potential far bigger than others). Most men nowhere near their possible structure. YOU can boost stature/posture/*presence* tenfold.

Aim for target YOU want whether to rid-fat/add-bulk/stay-course or go ALL way to Bodychamp proportions.

When you want

45–60* minutes exercise a day, three days weekly: MON/WED/FRI best (= weekend's rest). TUES/THURS/SAT (or other perms) all right if these only free days.

* = *times can vary from 15–20 minutes to 3 hours (for specialist. Many take 1–1½ hours due to rests between exercises. Older people take longer breaks.*

Keep up workouts. Each week/every week/without fail.

When only 2 days possible try one workout on MON, one FRI. If only 1 day possible use it. Use everything. The lot. Even night shift workouts in factory neon.

Best times: 7–8 at night (at least 1 hour after nosh, preferably 2). Or 3.30–5.30 in afternoon (same re lunch). Otherwise: when you can fit it in.

Try PEAK HOUR (everyone has one).

Take temperature every ½ hour for 3 days (under tongue: 2 minutes). Note when mercury always rises above normal mark (same time each day). This *is* peak hour. Choose 1 hour before temperature rise and 1 hour after (can be any time in 24 hours depending on your metabolism).

EVERYTHING you do in this 2 hours is THE best.

NEVER workout MON/TUES/WED/THURS/FRI/SAT/SUN. Muscles crumble to ruins after blitzing body with exercise. BUT they grow even faster as result (on the TUES/THURS/SAT between MON/WED/FRI) on rest days.

Note: muscles really DO crave to grow bigger/bigger/biggest for YOU. Prove it NOW by resisting them and *see* results.

(a) Stand sideways to wall. Press arm *hard* (from shoulder to fingertips) against wall for 3 minutes. Stand away. Let arm go. Muscle fibres just resisted raise limb to shoulder-level robot-wise.

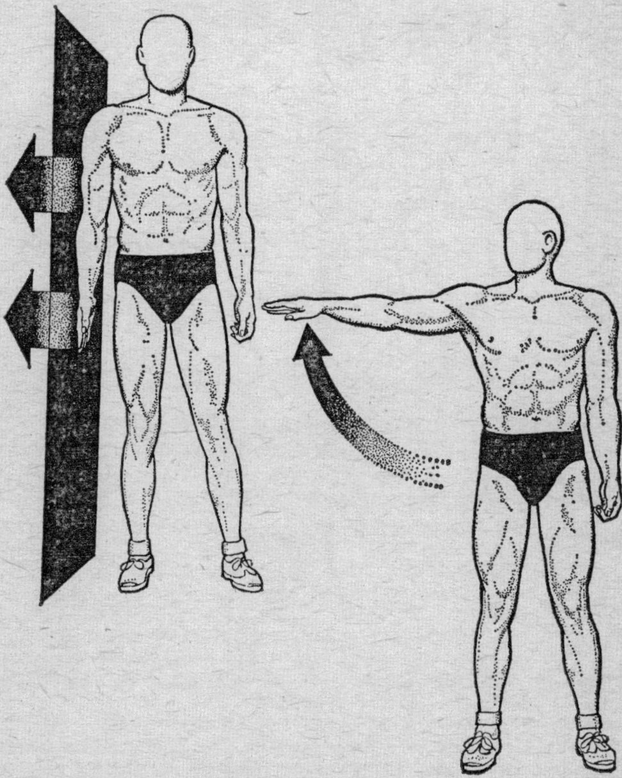

(b) Stand in narrow passage. Press hands palms reversed *hard* against walls for 3 minutes. Step out of passage. Letting arms go = arms rise as muscle fibres force against resistance (no longer there).

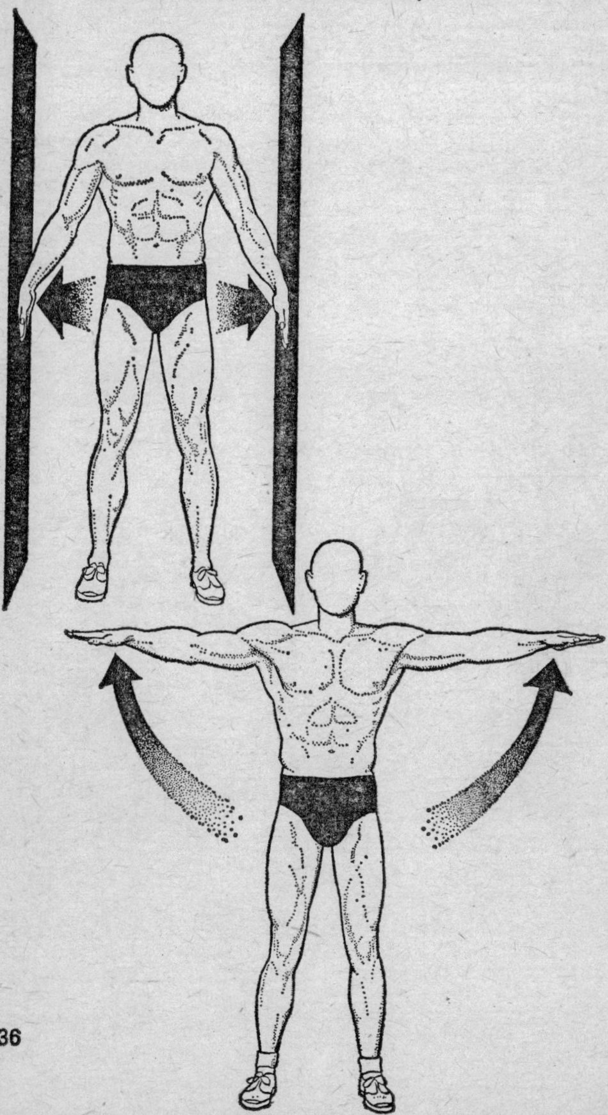

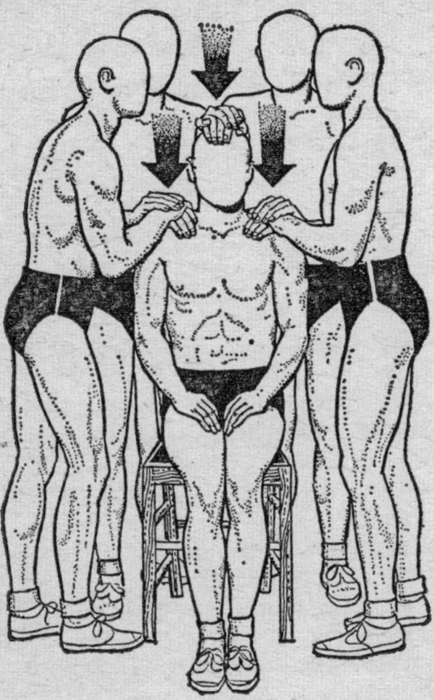

(c) Sit man on chair between 4 men. 4-non-sitters now PRESS all hands HARD on man's shoulders/head. After 3 minutes—GO ! Each places forefinger below *and* behind chair—which rises without effort (resisted muscles fighting back).

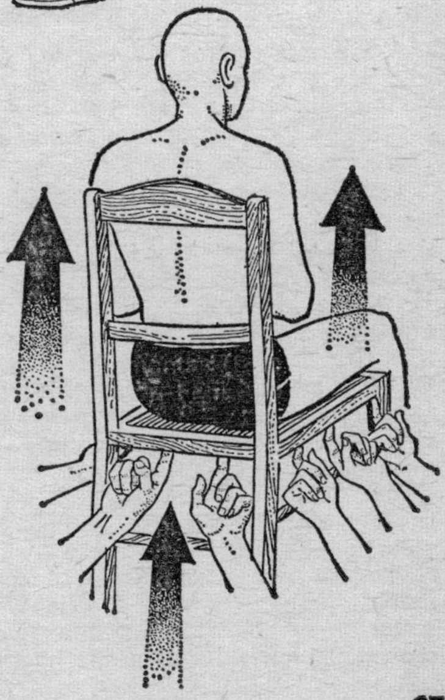

Muscles regroup power fast—bigger/stronger/tougher than before. You can FEEL this growth on off-days. No off-days = staleness/frustration/dark clouds.

Keep training. Don't lay off. Even keep in hand on holidays/business/duty. Reduced workout better than none. Only miss when unwell/tired (lazy?).

How you want

YOU choose own programme from rest of MR TOUGH.

1. MAKE LIST OF EXERCISES YOU PLAN TO DO (INCLUDING NO. OF REPS/SETS*).
2. GET FRIEND TO WORKOUT WITH YOU *IF* IT HELPS. ONE EXERCISES WHILE OTHER RESTS.
3. NEVER BEGIN WITH ADVANCED EXERCISES. BEGIN SLOWLY. PROGRESS STEADILY. DON'T OVERSTRAIN.
4. ONLY MAKE WORKOUTS HARDER AS BODY FINDS PRESENT ONES EASY.
5. DON'T EXPECT MUSCLES TO RIPPLE UP SUDDENLY. BUT EXPECT TO FEEL ROARING FIT.
6. WARM-UP FIRST WITH 5 MINUTE FITNESS FLEXERS USING EXERCISES CHOSEN FROM "FITTER IN A FORTNIGHT" TO CUT DOWN STRAIN/STIFFNESS.

** reps/sets = no. of times you do an exercise. Reps = revs. Sets = BURSTS of revs to let body have minute's breather in between (so blood can dose muscles). An exercise may have 30 reps done in 3 sets of 10. Thus = 3×10. May be more sets, may be less.*

Make muscles fight. Pit them v. odds. Push them hard. Squeeze out power. Milk the fibres. Piston/propel/wheel them into action. Smash down old muscle tissue, erect new each time muscles REALLY resisted.

WITH (as MR TOUGH shows) chairs/stools/tables. WITH books/brooms/rocks. WITH old iron. WITH scrap iron. WITH Iron-Game-Iron.* WITH sand bucket/gritty road/punchplank. WITH sandbags (stitch from 2 pieces 8"×14" canvas + 10 lbs. sand + 2 cord handles for ends). WITH rubber bands (2 old cycle inner tubes equally stretchy). WITH one limb push/push/pushing against another for 6 seconds (try to *pull* clasped hands apart counting 1001, 1002, 1003, 1004, etc.).

You pick. No 2 MR TOUGHS never toughen-up alike.

Some work fast. Some crawl. Some burn-off exercises galore. Some use only a few. Some handle BIG weights. Some the lightest. Some like ALL exercises. Some just one type—say weights (see below). Some don't even count reps (stop at predetermined muscle-shatter threshhold).

Fit pick into those 3 nights. Persevere. Make REAL effort. Keep to short regular sessions. Skip bombing muscles too savagely.

MR SOFT should follow reps/sets formula given with exercises. 8–12 reps with 3 sets generally best at first (later can vary a lot). Sometimes just 1 set enough at start.

NEVER struggle with heavy weights—whether extra tension in inner tubes (by looping extra rubber round hands) or adding too much iron to metal weights. Handle heaviest resistances you can do *in good style.*

Skip idea of doing 2 reps only but with GIANT load. Vital to do 8–10–12 reps with *manageable* load.

Remember: last TWO reps = golden charms of muscle-growing. Ensure YOU do them. In good style. With common sense resistance. THEY force-up muscle.

As MR TOUGH seems possible to YOU . . . increase resistances.

> * *Iron Game = weight training with sets/reps using below-maximum weights (NOT weight lifting which = bunking-up one massive weight in a contest). Scan muscle mag ads for different kits. Buy minimum gear. Add as you go. Share with mate. Initially needed: barbell (bar 5 or 6 feet long with 2 or more discs locked by collars—buy 5 ft. one if space short, 6 ft. one if room as more whip and far better); dumbells (have 14–18 in. rods and sleeve slides over rod as spacer and handgrip. Can be centrally loaded without sleeve to make swingbell gripped with both fists). All can have discs added from under 21 lbs. to 50 lbs. Much bigger gear range ready for YOU as power comes.*

Wind extra loop of inner tube round hands/quicken reps/add more to reps.

Find right iron weights for YOU by experiment over few days. Select weight which lets you do 8 reps where last 2 or 3 are hardest but possible with a fight. *And in good style.* Never sacrifice style for poundage. Add more weight when you can, as often as you can, as much as you can (up to 5 lbs.).

Know it makes sense to work with weights well below total lifting capacity. REPS do the good in Iron Game toughening (as in any exercise). Right resistance = smooth/no-jerk/electric performance.

Where you want

Where BODILY (taken for granted you have 7′+8′ air space to work in). Take care selecting BODY PARTS for toughening.

Some body parts a lot stronger than others (arms if docker; legs if pedestrian; fingers if spin bowler). Match other body sections with these. Don't get vain of one well-muscled slab and try to make it gigantic.

Pick out correct exercises to develop YOU all-round. Use routines you *need* to muscle-up NOT just ones you like.

Use imagination. Never exercise for toughness with one method (say favourite sport). Use that sport *and* several other ways. Football alone misses torso top. Tennis alone misses one arm. Swimming alone misses carrying muscles.

At first do reps/sets indicated (usually 8–12). Later mould own muscular destiny.

Strength/power/bulk = low reps + heavy weights (say 4–6 reps in 5–6 sets).

General development = medium reps + lighter weights (say 10 reps in 3 sets).

Endurance/slimness = high reps + light weights (say 15 or 20 reps).

REAL toughness = ALL body tempered/honed/stropped. Keep your cool over going wild about huge lats/great pecs/mighty arms to show off jacket . . . and neglect legs/backside/neck.

Rebuild body to robot standards: mechanically sound. Arm = jacknife with biceps spring to close blade, triceps spring to snap-out blade. Grease only biceps (with exercise) and rusty triceps snarl-up action. Other muscles pair up same way too.

Toughen-up ALL body.

So you ALWAYS want

Guard against never making it.

1. KEEP PROGRAMME VERY SIMPLE AT FIRST.
2. DON'T OVERCRAM WITH EXERCISES NOR OVERDO THEM.
3. KEEP EXERCISES EASY AT FIRST IF UNFIT.
4. CHANGE WORKOUTS EVERY 6–8 WEEKS.
5. DO HAVE A PLAN.

Muscles can be blitzed/bombed/shelled for 6–8 weeks (body grows in plateaux). Then it surrenders, muscles no longer recuperate. Staleness sets in.

Over-training is most insidious enemy of MR TOUGH. If anxious to make great gains = muscles do too much. So YOU no longer grow. No longer respond to workouts. Muscle pump packs up. Lactic acid builds up in tissues = muscle pain/discomfort. You go spongey, lack resilience. Anxiety follows.

Get in first. Take a change not a layoff. For 2 weeks on plateau brink—do group of new/unusual/random exercises. Attack body zones from new angle. Do 1–2 sets with 8–12 reps. Try out NEW approach.

After 2 weeks go back to old routine with new slant. Pick different exercises to attack same muscles from fresh slants. Get more "style" with new muscle growth over next 6–8 weeks.

During 6–8 week change (lasting 2 weeks) only work muscles enough to keep in tone. Change diet—new, tasty meals, fresh fruits, juices, etc. Go all out for new ideas/scene/body.

Other staleness (if off-colour/jaded/mixed-up elsewhere) = miss out on FRI session (if MON/WED/FRI man). Layoff raises steam for the next MON.

GIVE IT ALL YOU'VE GOT

Body and soul (nothing but).

Body

Forget fresh-air nut-case image. Live strength silently. Keep toughness aim to self. Follow own image of power. Live up to it. In good clothes/shoes/haircut (buy fewer but better).

Don't act tough (talking from mouth corner/street corner/bar corner). Smile. Look smart. Have quiet calm coming from secret workouts. Know *the* power ticking over inside.

POWER from V-forming torso. Deepening chest. Growing back. Thickening shoulders. Cuff-link-bursting wrists. Bone-crushing-fists. Flattening stomach. Tougher legs. Bronzing complexion. Straighter posture. Better wind. Added cool.

Slot tougheners into between-workout days.

Lug dustbins to gate (each hand palm up, bending elbow 5 reps each arm). Jump for low tree branches and chin up a few reps. Carry objects (like books) in hands, raise out to shoulder level like wings (and *hold*). Dig garden. Mow lawn (loads of arm movement). Pump arms back/forwards (elbows right back). Grip shave-foam aerosol as if to mash metal.

Use each weekend for tough project. Rock climb. Canoe rapids. Plumb pothole. Swim tarn/river/lake. Sail. Row. Skin dive. Water-ski. Parachute. Hill-walk. Hike. Orienteer. Ski. Run. Pony trek. Skate. Chop trees. Chip logs. As MR TOUGH will show.

Soul (especially subconscious).

Be excited about becoming strong. Enthuse enthusiasm. Aim high. Begin new era. Search for adventure. Be inspired/absorbed/gripped with strength ideal.

KNOW you are *bound* to gain real muscle with work. All men can pack power/punch/pull. 18 months from now = Titan/Goliath/Samson very certainly emerging from YOU.

Quest strength. Visit gyms. Strong men shows. PE courses. Send for free literature of strength appliances to *interest*-interest. Read all on toughness (from novel GEORDIE to muscle mags MR UNIVERSE/MUSCLE BUILDER/ALL-BRITISH ATHLETE). Eat/breathe/sleep power.

Never follow same old exercises year after year. Try all. Experiment in 2-weekly periods (between 6–8 weekly regular body plateau sessions). Select and reject.

Keen interest tones subconscious strength-motivated radar. New things on power skyline register with big bleep. And you try it. From now. . . .

TOES/FEET

TOES/FEET: 2

YOUR FEET were beautifully engineered. Bridges of bone/ arches of muscle/gussets of ligament incorporate weight distribution and suspension solutions to pack a week's computer programme.

Propping 12-stone man on pedestal capable of standing 700 lbs.-a-step-thrust; propelling YOU ¼-million miles through life; powerful-enough-weapon to smash into oppressor with 30 m.p.h. poke, feet were precision-honed.

But what ARE they now? Mechanical failures from misuse? Blubber stamps (which = clog-styled footprints on bathroom floor instead of shoe-shaped ones) from neglect? Track foot fitness first—and let MR TOUGH take over.

Make weak arms strong with footpower

In climbing a thick rope (feeblest man *can* using feet as propellant-aid). Climbing sequence = reach; rope grip with hands; tow upknees; TRAP ROPE WITH FEET; push legs straight; race fists up rope; rope grip with hands etc. Rope trap for feet is shown.

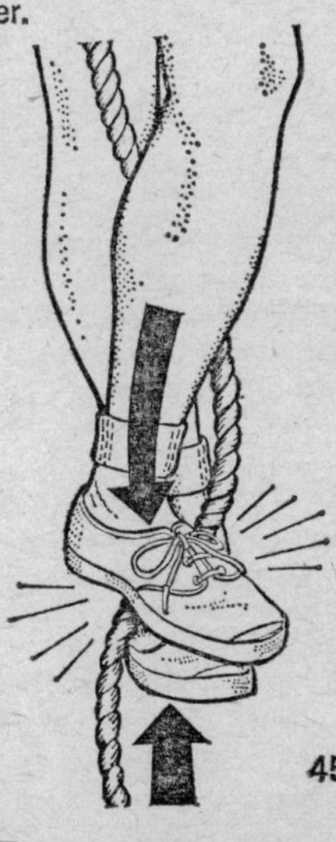

Defend YOURSELF

Your Leg is a survival self-defence weapon. Use when possible (longer reach/stronger than arm).

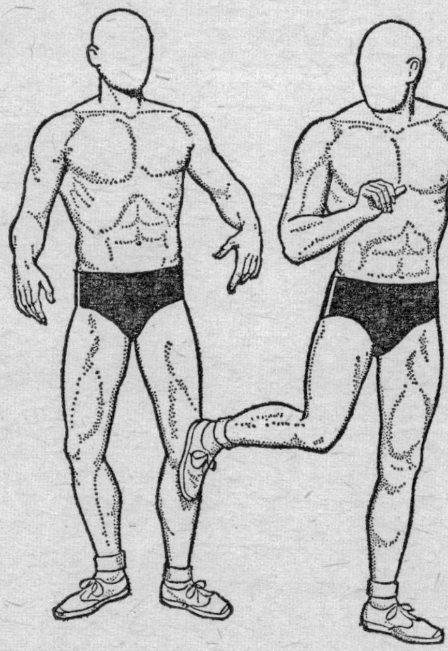

NEVER kick with the toe. (Foot easily avoided/grasped). Swivel on foot ball. Bend knee at same time. Drive heel of other foot backwards. Practise (with both feet). Blow = hard to stop (can be used at distance when opponent's arms still out of range). Go for his knee.

Use toes as skyhooks

In stockinged feet (grab like a crab on wet rock face). 16-stone man rockclimbs purely through toe power (and footedge). Get *guide/course/climber-mate* to rope YOU up roadside stoneface among vapour trails, wet ferns, aerocamera views, quartz crystals. Keep heels down, knees off rock. Use toes more than hands.

Wear pumps on dry rock.

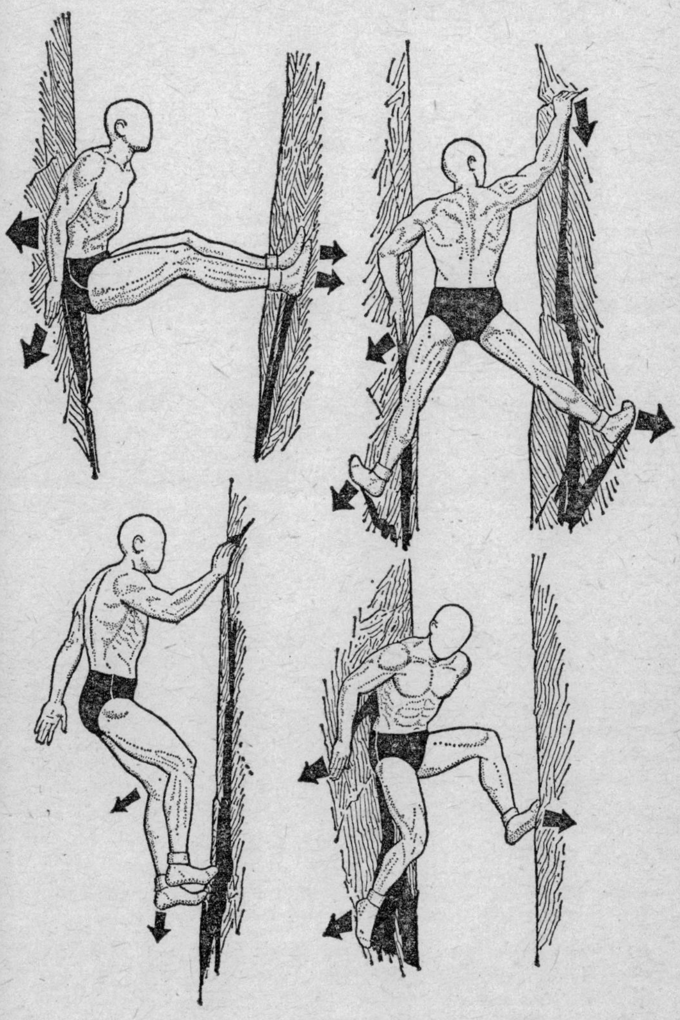

GET BEST OUT OF YOUR FEET AT ONCE

YOUR FEET are earthmoving levers. Just look at mechanical advantages going for MR TOUGH from these Herculean struts.

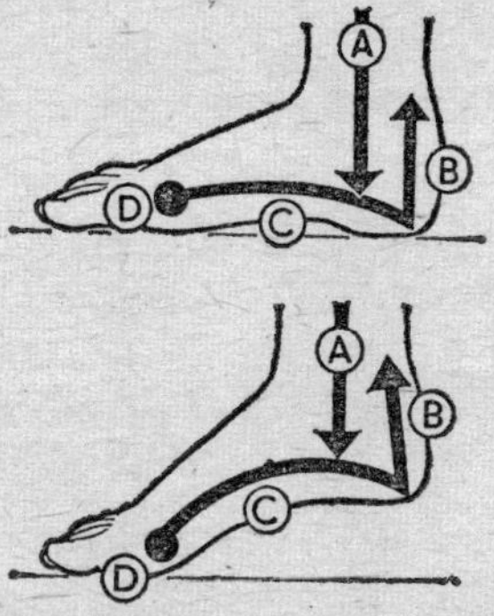

A = body weight forcing down.
B = lifting power through Achilles tendon from gastros.
C = long arched lever of foot which pivots about. . . .
D = foot fulcrum (formed by metatarsal heads).

OR as they look X-rayed.

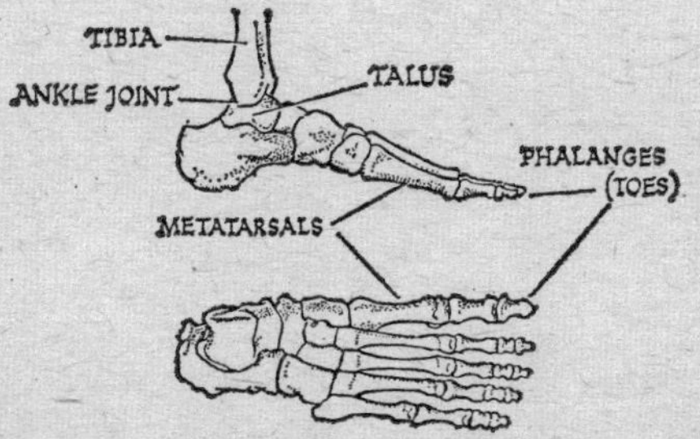

Treat feet right to-day. And.

Every day

Wash feet daily in warm water. Plunge into cold. Do brisk rub with thorny towel. Dry carefully between toes. Swap socks each day.

NEVER whip off icy shoes and thaw feet on hot pipes (chilblain risk). Nylon socks OUT if YOU have cold feet (use thick wool). IF persistently freezing feet—see Dr (for confirmation it is NOT Raynaud's disease/anaemia/lumbago).

Swab with surgical spirit (never pickle to toughen = bad

blister potential). Dust lightly with talc/foot powder/baby powder.

Cut toe nails straight across. Never curved or slanting.

Every night
Keep feet warm for vital sleep (+ extra blankets if needed). Wearing socks = one answer. Keep boots out of sleeping bags.

Everybody
See chiropodist if bad corns/hammer toe/ingrowing toenails. Or toes which ride on top of neighbour. Or prominent heels, elevated 5th toe, bunions, bad athlete's foot, sprains/fractures/strains. Or if you waddle.

Sort out flat feet *now*.

If wet footprints bulge out *both* sides get chiropodist check to see HOW bad. Flat feet causing aches/bad posture/back troubles are 3-staged.

(a) Foot arch there when you sit BUT sinks as you stand. Curable. Practice walking toes-in. Do this daily . . . rise on tiptoe, roll feet outwards to edges, stand so weight comes down edges, turn feet in. 20 reps a time (*see later*).

If standing all day change job. Never have everything at hand during work: *walk* to reach it. Pacing MUCH better than standing. If overweight—reduce fast.

(b) When arch is flat even at rest BUT can still be shaped with hands—slight hope. Arch supports probably needed in shoes to prop up inner side of heel/sole. Possibly physiotherapy too.

(c) Final stage = rigid flat foot (unbendable). Little to be done. If no muscular pain feet best left alone. *Can* sometimes be improved by orthopaedic surgeon manipulating foot.

Everywhere
Wear socks inside-out (smoother to feet).

When blister-risk from new boots/shoes/clogs smear agricultural soap (soft soap) on to sock innards. As footballers do.

Bandaid bandage minus lint dressing = another blister stopper. Stick it on any slightly sore heel well *before* skin chafes.

Never prick blisters (dry-elastoplast them).

Wash/air feet when possible through day in hot weather. Washing in cold water is excellent body reviver.

Beat foot cramp by hand-bending toes towards shin as soon as twinge felt. Knead with fingers until hardness goes.

Every foot
Out of 200 million shoes sold in Britain yearly half were wrong size (right-handers usually = right feet at least ½ size bigger than left feet). Remember. . . .

Always have shoes fitted personally. Working shoes need to

be best fit of all. Try *both* shoes of a pair. Have feet measured when standing (toes spread). Shoe-shop around mid-day as feet swell 5 per cent when walking.

Shoes fit best when . . .

1. BIG TOE MISSES TIP AS YOU STAND.
2. SHOE HEEL HUGS OWN HEEL SNUGLY.
3. SIDES DO NOT GAPE.
4. LITTLE TOES LIE FLAT IN EACH SHOE.

Buy best quality shoes you can (last longer/treat feet/look good). 2 or 3 pairs needed so shoe-swap possible each day (foot moisture needs to dry out). Plastic shoe trees train shoes to MR TOUGH'S shape.

Bunions/corns/calouses best battled with shoes having: soft lining; smooth inside seams; stitching not too close to edges; pliable, durable materials; reputable trade mark.

TOUGHEN-UP FEET DAILY

Tougher feet = marvellous feeling. See doctor for a tetanus injection NOW and begin.

Harden soles

Go walks/runs barefooted. Leave shoes/socks behind. Flat foot it (forcing *all* of feet on to ground). Don't chicken out and tiptoe over gravel, etc. Forget grit/dogmuck/snails in dark (BUT know route in day to miss smashed glass, etc.). Press on to win feet of iron (*not* flappy/squelchy/horrible things). Feet *feel* velvet-toned.

Get sun/air/water often to feet. Kick beachball bare-instepped. Dribble small sandbag naked-toed. Wash car shoeless. KNOW this = *real* foot toughening.

Train bones

Many foot exercises risky. BUT two excellent for children/adults of most foot conditions.

1. STAND FOOT PLANTED FIRM.

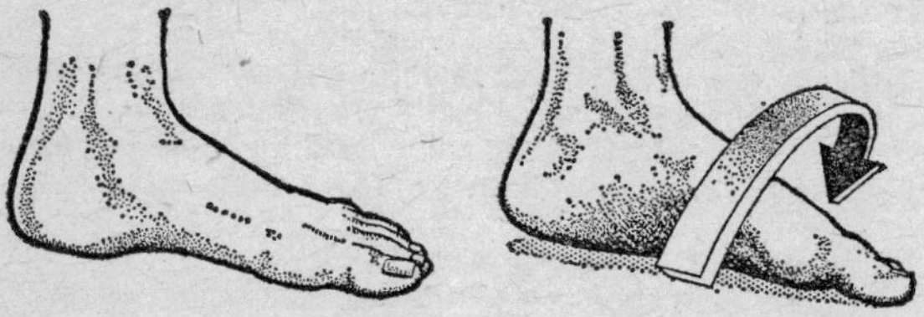

2. ROLL WHOLE FOOT ON TO OUTER BORDER SO SOLE FACES IN A BIT.

3. HOLD THIS POSITION AND ...

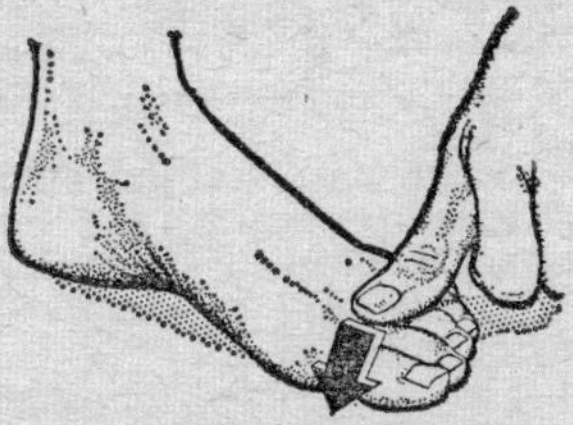

4. FORCE BALL OF FOOT ON THE FLOOR.
5. KEEP DOING THIS OFTEN.

*= *foot ball forcing may need thumb pressure at first.*

Other exercise best shown by *hand* action.

Press hands flat on table. Force down hand heels and finger pads to force knuckles up off surface. Knuckles arch = similar one in foot. So . . .

1. STAND FOOT ROOTED SOLID.
2. PRESS DOWN TOE PADS TO FORCE FOOT "KNUCKLES" UP.

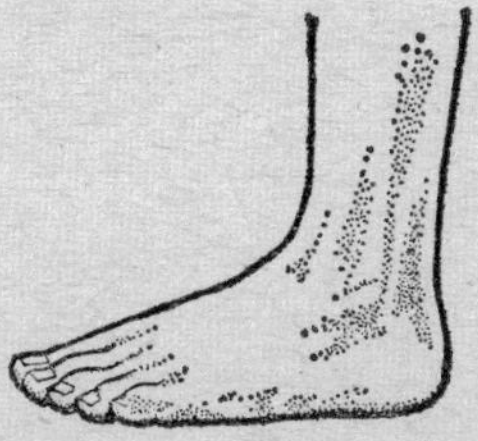

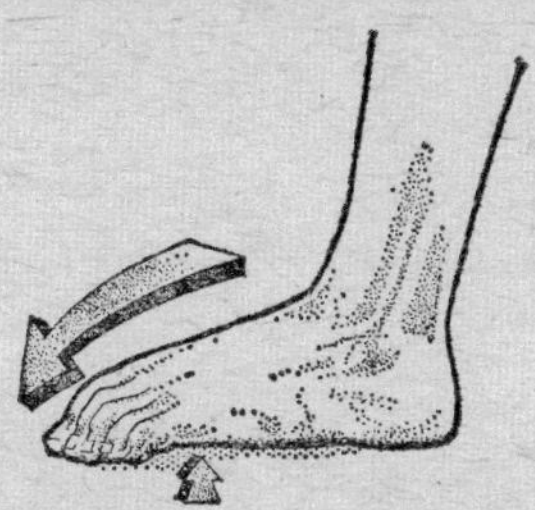

Easier if toes overlap book edge $\frac{1}{2}$ in. thick. Do it often while shaving, etc.

IF feet in fair fettle try other barefoot exercises through day—especially if overweight/standing on the job.

Choose from these:

(a) Sit and shake ankles with feet totally relaxed.

(b) Walk on heels (toes pointing front) across room and back 2 or 3 times.

(c) Lean on wall and stand feet just astride, toes to front. Raise heels as high as possible and lower. 20 reps.

(d) Sit on chair and do alternate foot raises off floor, rotating ankle outwards, pointing toes. Do 5 reps out then 5 reps in with each foot. In 3–5 sets.

(e) Sit with one leg across knee, grasp heel with one hand and upper part of foot with other. Twist foottop until you see sole (holding heel fast). 5 reps a foot.

(f) Sit on chair, feet flat on floor, toes to front. Lift toes-only up to spread them then lower. And toe-grab 3d. bit/marble/ballpoint off floor. 5 reps.

(g) Sit on chair with feet just apart, toes front. Rub sole of right foot on left foot instep in clockwise movement. And vice versa. 10 reps a foot.

(h) Stand feet just astride holding table. Rock forward on toes and back on heels (lift toes high on rock-back). 20 reps.

LEGS

LEGS: 3

YOUR LEGS are YOUR roots. Sucking up rockcracking power from tone-up toil they gird your trunk with girth of an oak/husk of a chestnut/resilience of a mountain ash. And GROW and GROW while planting you firm.

Dig those roots into surging leg exercises NOW for thighs to make a pine tree jealous. And for TREETOP chest/shoulders potential too (leg graft = TOTAL bodybuilding with *strong* breathing + *good* blood pumping).

Are YOU still a beanstalk? You will never find big branches on puny trunks nor might trunks on feeble roots. Start rooting for MR TOUGH to-day with rugged leg exercise to burndown/regrow muscle like a forestfire.

WHAT YOUR LEGS CAN DO AT ONCE

YOU are as strong as YOUR legs (most powerpacked muscles in body here).

Lift a BIG man from the deck

Start on 10 stone men first. Then work up.

IF using *both* hands bend down (as shown) until hands can clasp behind man's small of back.

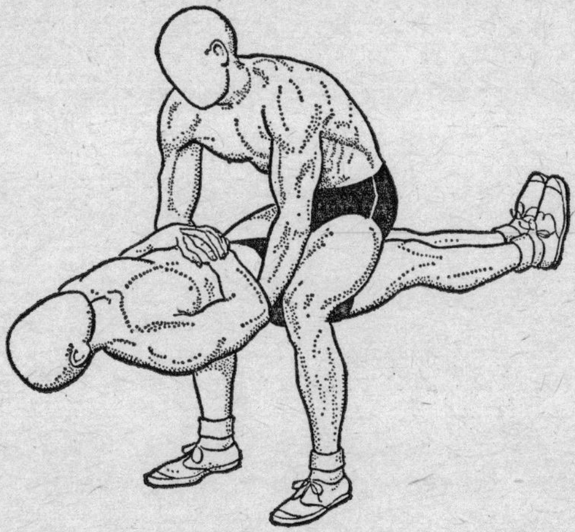

1. GET READY, BENDING KNEES.
2. THINK ONLY OF STRAIGHTENING LEGS.*
3. HYDRAULIC–POWER THOSE LEGS STRAIGHT...
4. UNTIL KNEES LOCK AND...
5. MAN IS OFF FLOOR.

*= *again, only leg power (and back strength) lifts. Arms simply used as cables.*

(see also NECK)

IF using one arm only:

1. STOOP/BEND KNEES/GRASP MAN'S BELT BUCKLE WITH FIST.
2. FORGET PULLING WITH ARMS.
3. REMEMBER PUSHING WITH LEGS.

And lift man 12 in. from deck to prove point.

Shove/push/heave more easily
Again POWER comes from *legs.* Whether lifting boxes/pushing cars/carrying logs.

NEVER jerk, strain or wrestle at rupturepoint. Breathe freely. Act smoothly. Concentrate on leg power. Use arms/shoulders/ back as *secondary* forces.

Push bogged mini-van thus...

1. FACE BACKDOORS GRIPPING ROOF-RIM WITH ...
2. ARMS/LEGS/BODY IN DEAD STRAIGHT LINE.
3. LOCK ELBOWS.
4. SHOVE HORIZONTALLY AND FORWARD NOT UPWARD.
5. DRIVE/DRIVE/DRIVE FROM LEGS.

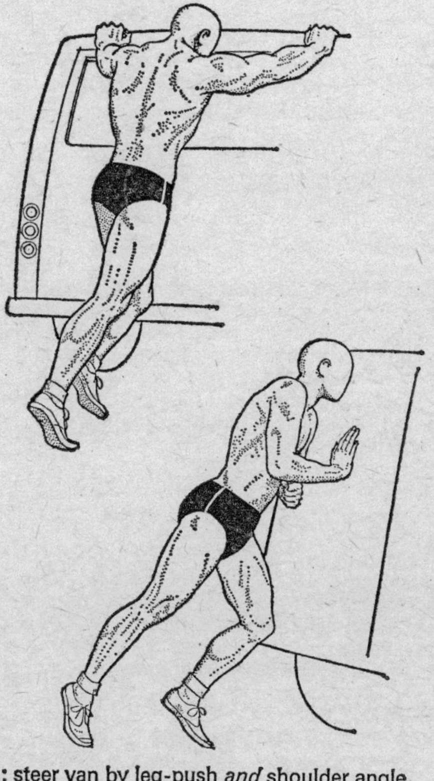

Note: steer van by leg-push *and* shoulder angle.
(see also SHOULDERS/BACK)

Swim as never before
By using legs the REAL way.

BUOYANT BREASTSTROKE = NOT being propelled by legs/arms together. Make alternate strokes: legs towards body as arms pull back; legs push back as arms go forward. Keep it constant. Leg movement = nonwide kickback (NEVER dangling down). Straighten floating body with downward narrow armpull (NOT wide).

GREAT CRAWL = NOT using feet as propellors. Slow down. Only show heels above water (do NOT kick spray). Keep legs dead straight as they kick up/down. Paddle one foot then other driving down 18 in. from hip. End each legstroke with downward ankle twist. Body follows legs example—ALL straight. Arms going straight ahead in water slowly/strongly (point palms away from body, thumb down). An arm pulls through until hanging vertically down: then pushes to thigh.

BATTLING BACKSTROKE = sub-aqua knees (ALL time). Only toes must break surface. DO 6 leg movements to each complete action of arms (which brush ears). As one arm ends its downward motion other arm should cut into water.

Walk tall

Up Snowdon/Ben Nevis/Mont Blanc tracks. Try local hill first for powerscene revelation.

Tortoisepaced. Flatfooted (boots clamped down). Eyes down. keepingoing. Rythmic-striding. Nonresting. Boot toes turning to next-step-direction. Short-stepping. Rock/tussock/boulder skimming. Zigzagging up steeps. Never tiptoeing. Leaning forward a bit.

Note: jam heel on pebble/stone/bump at every chance. And concentrate on thighmuscle thrust by *locking* each leg in turn behind knee (stiff/straight).

WATCH KNEES

Vulnerable leg zones. Cosset/pad/protect against potential pressure.

Sharp kneecap pain CAN KO you. Body heat escapes HERE in bitter chill (and can = hypothermia to jeanwearers on mountains). Housemaid's Knee happens to toughest potholers *if* knees used too much in cave crawling.

Kneel easy. Pad with towel in toneups involving knee pressure. Keep them off rocks climbing/caving/camping.

DAILY LEG TONING

Walk-run up hills/stairs/sand dunes. Longterm limbering = heman posture/wildcat stamina/rhino power. Start coming on NOW with regular daily sessions. Or make it alternate days (as for Iron Game). Tryout toners. See which are YOU.

Experiment first. Find regular programme depending on wants/needs/urge. *And* condition. Do as many/few as YOU decide. Then . . . don't chop/change day by day.

Note: fit can skip toners and head for POWER producers with hard resistance to muscles. Check fitness score (see BODY).

Bicycling
Shoulders on floor. Hips/legs roof-pointing. Small of back/glutes hand-supported. Pedal legs in small circle.* HARD *and* FAST but never for TOO LONG. Reps to enoughs-enough point (with extra 2 for luck).

*= *bring knees down lowest on UP stroke.*

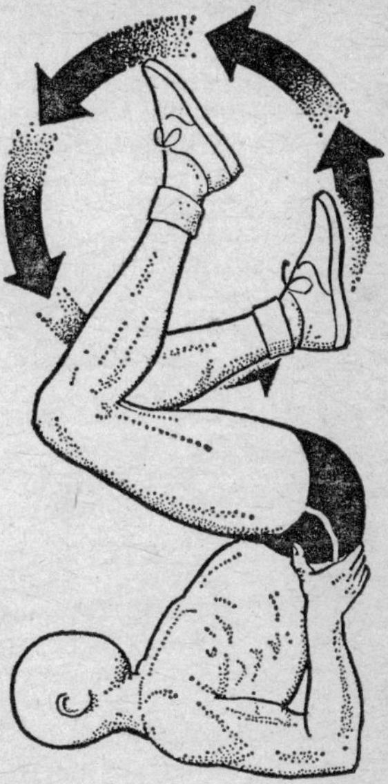

Deep knee bends
Stand feet foot apart. Relax. Count 1. Sink down until thighs parallel to floor (hands on hips or behind neck or straight out for balance). Keep eyes dead ahead, back straight.

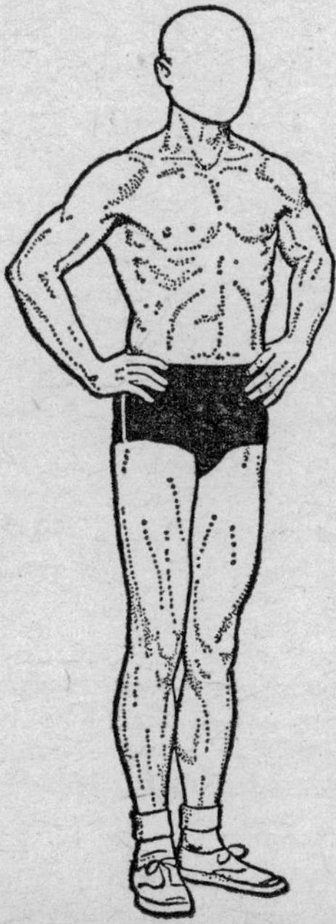

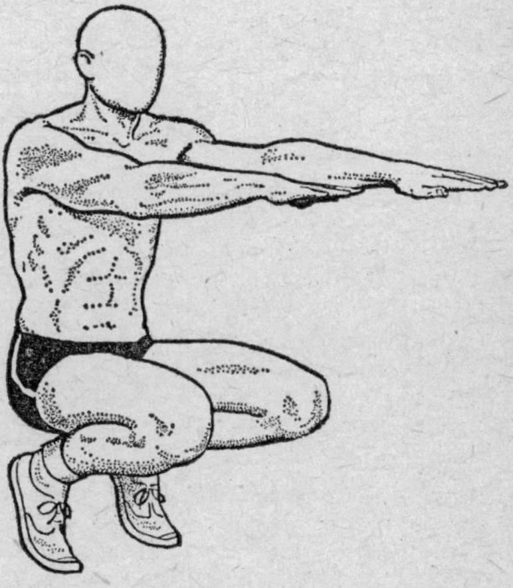

Count 2. Return to vertical breathing out. 5–10 reps withslow buildup to 25.
Note: NOT a flatfooted toner; use feetballs.

Step ups (see also BODY)
Up/down on kitchen chair standing straight (arms to side). Start with ½ minute routine. Then expand time/speed up rep rate.

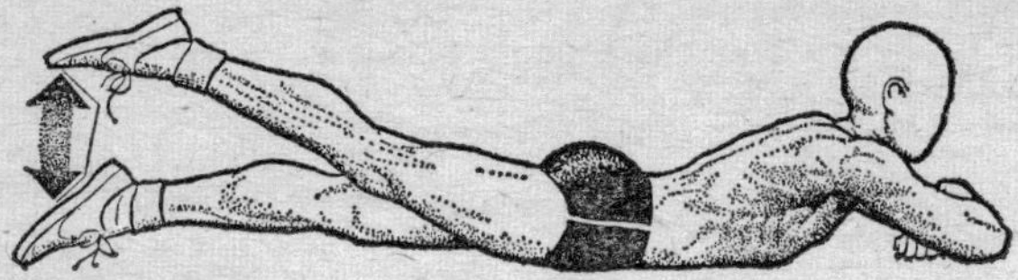

Prone leg kicking
Lie prone as shown. Lash back straightlegged and UP. Reps to enough's-enough.

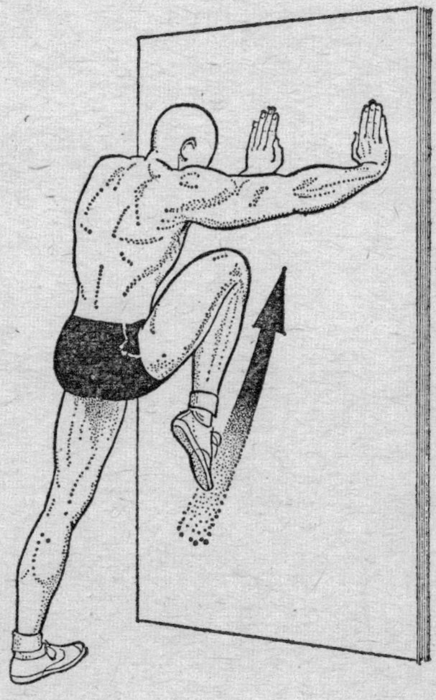

Knees ups
Push on wall leaning body forward straightlined from heels–shoulders. Haul knee to chest then swap *rapidly* machinegun style.

Clamp down heel of leg support. 25 reps a leg.

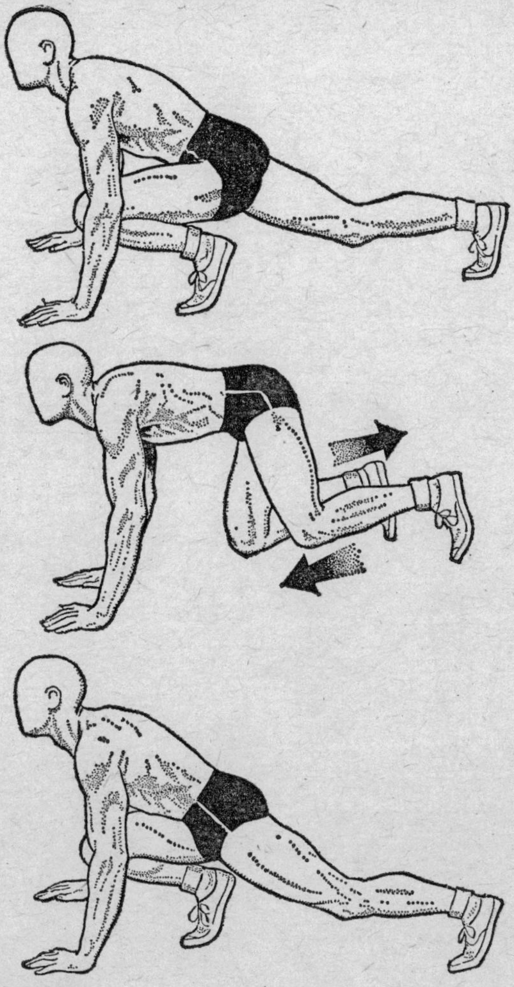

Knee pump
Balance weight on hands/toes AND piston knees by shooting one leg back while firing other forward at fastlick.

10 reps a day for 14 days, 15 reps for 3rd week, 20 reps thereafter until maximum of 25 possible. Will wind MR SOFT so easy/easy/easy at first.

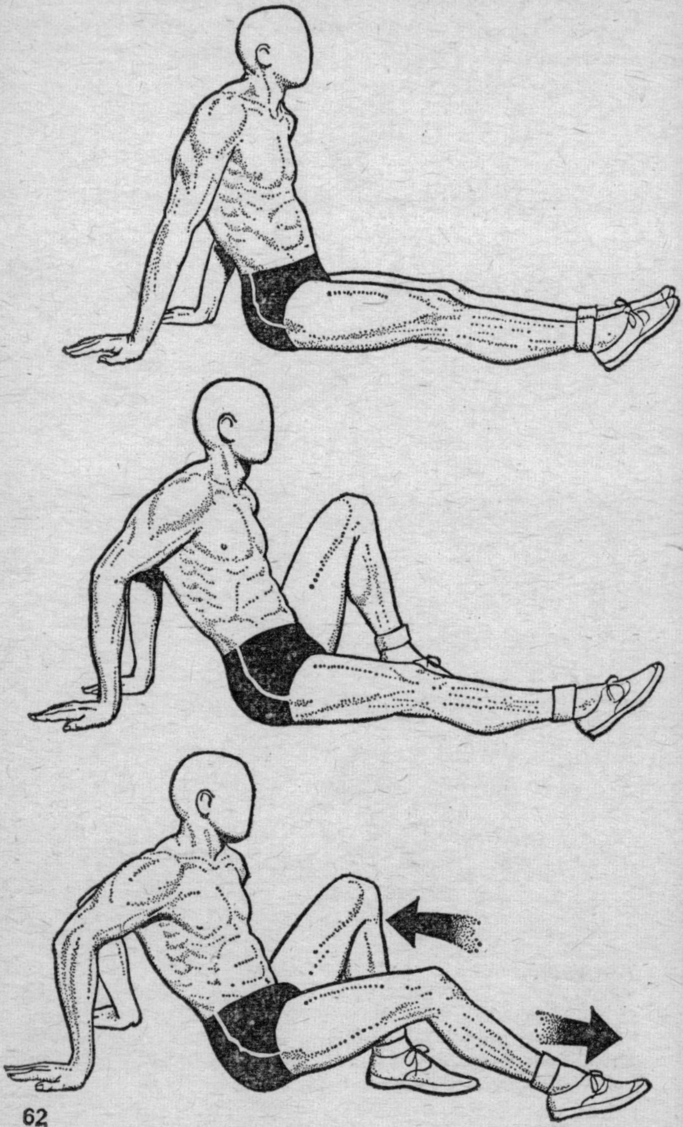

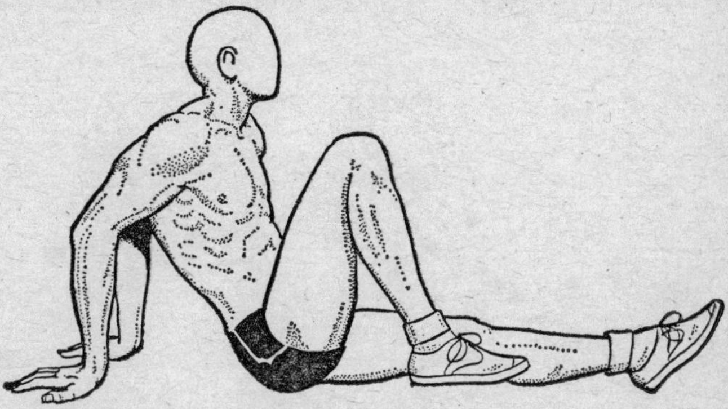

Seated knee pump

HARD.

Sit on floor and kick out knees. Lifting action needed which takes weight of whole leg on thighs/hips. Snap one knee at a time HIGH for chest. Swap legs (pumping first with one, then other).

10 reps a leg first week, 12 second and 15 after that. No more than 25 ever.

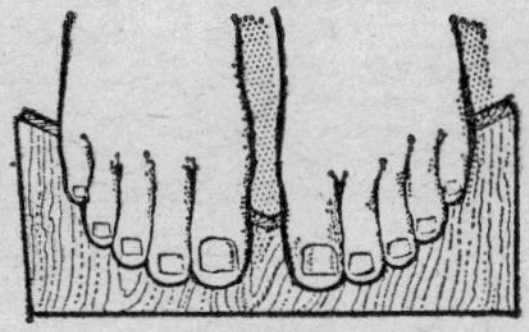

Toe risers

Prop toes on 3 in. plank/book/step. Lock legs straight and together. Point toes at 90 degrees. Tiptoe UP with straight legs, hands on hips, eyesahead. Slowly. And *lower* slower. 25 reps feet parallel; then 25 reps heels pointing out; then 25 reps toes out. This = 75 reps. Workup to 50 in each position.

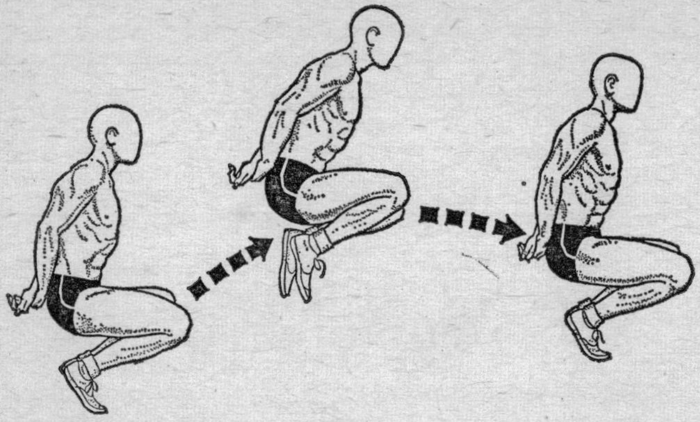

Rabbit hopping

HARD.

Clasp hands behind back. Bend knees. Lower hips. And stand on toes. Bound up and forward for 10 yards. Work up to 50.

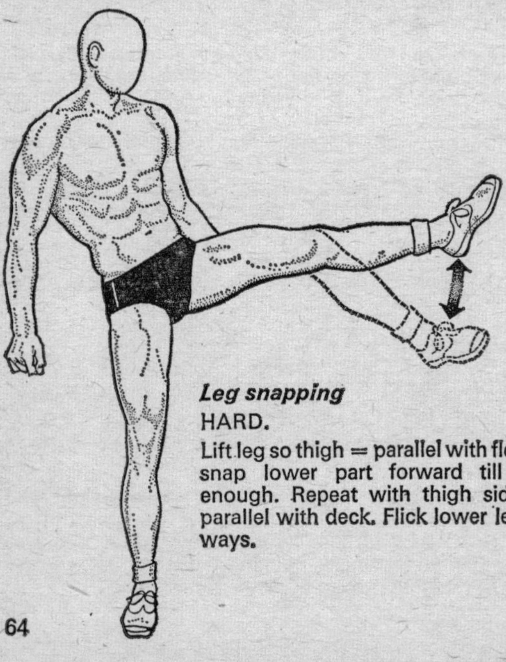

Leg snapping

HARD.

Lift leg so thigh = parallel with floor. Sharply snap lower part forward till enough's-enough. Repeat with thigh sideways and parallel with deck. Flick lower leg out sideways.

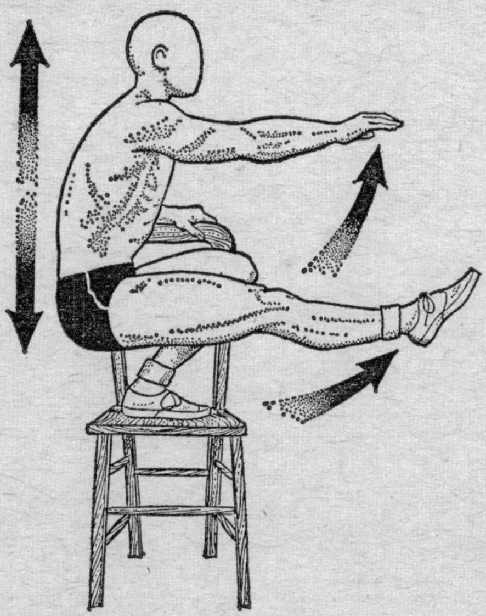

Russian knee bend

HARD.

Place back of chair near supporting wall. Stand on chair with left leg near back (grip this lefthanded). Raise right arm and leg and *slowly* sink to 4-knee bend on chair. Keep heel clamped to seat (propup heel with book if difficulty here). Right arm/leg MUST be raised until parallel/horizontal. Movement ends with knee bend completion.

10 reps with right leg, 10 with other (or working up to these targets). Work up to 25 each leg. Later weight can = book held in outstretched hand as resistance.

Squats with broomstick

1. STAND FEET JUST OVER FOOT ASTRIDE.
2. GRASP BROOM HANDLE ACROSS SHOULDERS.
3. CHIN UP/BACK STRAIGHT/LOOKING UP.
4. TAKE DEEP BREATH AND . . .
5. SINK TO DOUBLE KNEES BEND (CLAMPING FEET TO FLOOR).
6. STRAIGHTEN LEGS BREATHING OUT.

(see diagram overleaf)

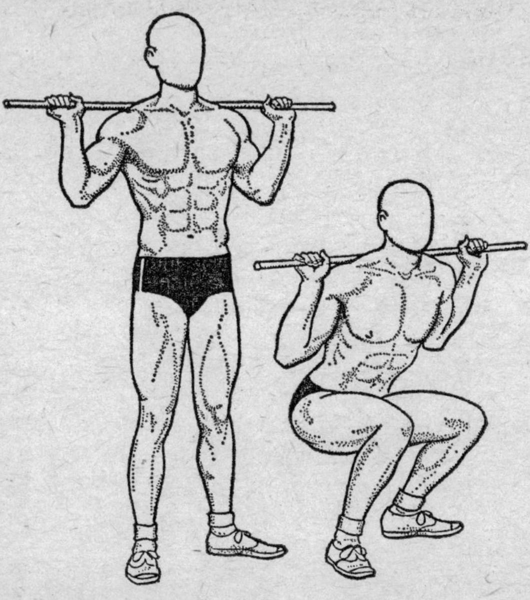

Note: mouth-breathing best for lungs/heart.

20 reps. Rest 5 minutes. Do 20 more. Rest another 5. Do final 20 reps.

Keep easy/steady rhythm—NO rush. Turn toes out if heels keep rising (knack is soon learnt).

INSTANT MICROPOWERING

6 seconds an exercise daily whenever YOU want. Pick YOUR own series (swing changes monthly).

Doorway developers

(a) Stand in doorway with back/head pressing against one jamb, one foot forced flat on the other jamb. Breathe in. PUSH foot HARD (6 seconds).

(b) Reach up to push lintel both-handed arms straight. *Legs bent.* Standing on box (if needed). TRY to jack up legs and push lintel through roof (6 seconds).

(c) Stand in doorway centre back to a jamb. Raise left heel 8 in. off floor and force back against jamb. Do 6 second kickback nonmoving. Swap feet.

(d) Stand in mid-doorway facing out. Lift right foot sideways until halted by jamb. Lock legs straight and PUSH sideways (6 seconds). Swap feet.

(e) Close door. Slouch on it hands pocketed. Force back with legs when half sitting/standing for 6 seconds.

Chair toners

(a) Sit with feet flat on floor (heels against chair legs). FORCE back with heels (6 seconds).

(b) Sit stretching out legs with ankles crossed. Lock one foot solid behind other. Order brain to rip them apart BUT hold foot position for 6 seconds. Swap over ankles.

(c) Flex legs (drawing back under chair seat). Sit up. Lock one foot over other. Securely. Order brain to part feet. Keep strain up for 6.

(d) Sit crossing ankles so lower foot is FLAT on floor. Order brain to yank back forward foot (blocked by anchored ankle). 6 seconds pressure.

(e) Stand by chair feet astride. Order brain to close legs. Battle against order-pressure for 6.

(f) Close legs and reverse order. Frustrate leg parting motions for 6 HARDFOUGHT seconds.

Floor conditioners

(a) Sit on floor one leg out (locked at knee). Hug other knee bent double. *Tug back* toes/foot of outstretched limb for 6 seconds. Swap legs/feet/toes.

(b) Ditto. BUT point toes away of kneelocked limb for 6 second stretch. Swap toes.

(c) Sit on floor feet drawn up until legs bent at 90 degrees. Wrap doubled towel round/across ankles. Grip ends. Yank HARD against brainorder to straighten legs: 6.

(d) Lie back on floor. Flex knee so lower leg parallel to floor. Loop towel round footsole. Fight straight leg-brainorder nonmoving for 6.

(e) Sit on floor both legs straight out. Run towel across feet balls. Pull taut so feet come vertical. Try pointing toes versus towelpull for 6.

(f) Floorsit gripping wooden chair legs with ankles of outstretched legs. Balance with handpalms on floor. And try to CRUSH chair for 6.

(g) Weight down chair seat (with books etc.). Floorsit in front. Lock one foot instep under chair seat edge. *Both* legs straight. FIGHT to kickup chair for 6.

USE IRON POWER

MON/WED/FRI routine with weights CAN = steel trap poise/

naplam muscle wrap/explosive POWer.

Use SQUAT as THE essential powerbuilder in book (reasons later). Include one thigh bicep grafter (say thigh curl in boots/or with mate). Other powerpackers like leg split/lateral legraise + iron boots/etc. = optional extras. Don't pack routine with too much.

Calf muscles = VERY tough. Pile work on them. Never neglect lower legs. Use, say, 2 heel raising exercises (straddle jumping/heel raises/donkey raises) WITH the toe raise exercise.

REMEMBER: training IS individual. Can differ vastly between people. Start slowly. Pick few MAIN exercises at first—then branch out.

Generally: highish poundages + fewish reps = BEST for Oxfam Ad types (easily exhausted); high reps + lots of work = BEST for Michelin Men (who can AFFORD to burn up more energy unlike the skinny).

After 6–8 weeks have 2 weeks to experiment with new exercises for NEXT 6–8 weeks (see BODY). Do bodyparts in same order second 6–8 week session BUT drop at least half. Substitute new powerpackers from choice below to hit muscles from new angles. Do same *every* 6–8 weeks.

Perm variety of exercises each 6–8 week periods. Do it 3 ways: cut out present/fetch in new/bring back old. Right through YOUR ironmanmaking career.

POWERPACK THIGHS

Tapemeasure round thickest part of legtop (keeping tape level). BEST test = slimline pants musclepacked-firm.

Squats

THE real McKoy.

And most vital (plus most hated) powerpacker to build up MR TOUGH. NEVER be a crybaby over squats (even thinnest man can hope to tote 200 lbs. plus in squats ultimately). Nor neglect squats for showy lat/delt/bicep exercises. SQUATS = best of THE 3 main body conditioners (see also bench press/deadlift). NEVER move to day's squat dose with bowed head. Lift it high and....

REALISE squats do NOT weaken/kill/discomfort YOU if done properly; need YOU to set YOURSELF for mighty effort before taking barbell off stand;* must have YOU gearedup mentally before the action; need deliberate nonrush technique. THEN ... bar will lose weight; YOU will fly through reps.

Diag. 147

*** = buy squat racks so you can back under load (under £10 a pair) or make from iron gaspipe (barrel) + scrap metal. 1 in. inside diameter pipe will make either type**

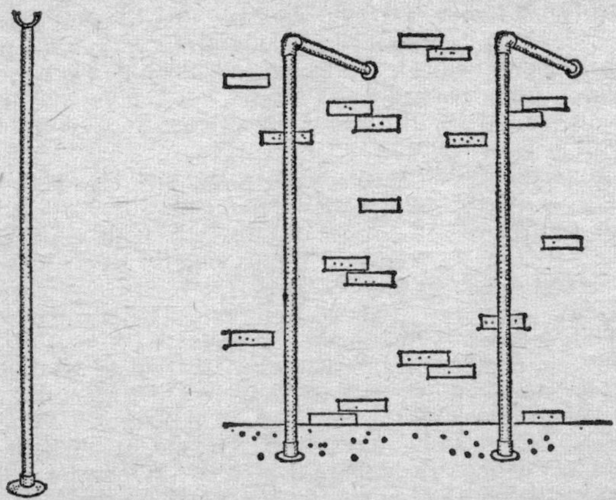

A or B as shown (ironmongers will thread pipe for you). Uprights = 4 ft long.

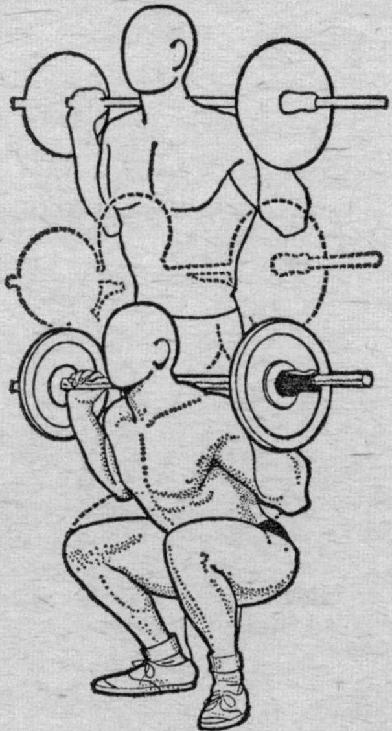

SQUAT movement = same as with broomstick (see earlier). Keep back flat. Incline torso slightly forward from waist. Tyros best to do only half-squats first 2–3 weeks (thighs only go as far as parallel with floor: no further). PAUSE only briefly at bottom (NEVER bounce back straight up).

Inhale deeply before legs are bent; breathe out as you push up.

REMEMBER: use weights YOU can just about handle so you have to fight over *last 2 reps.* Showing off with too heavy weights = terrible error.

General fitness = 3 or 4 sets of 15–20 reps. Up to 30.
Real leg power = 3 to 5 sets of 5–6 reps.
Stamina/power = 3 sets of 5 reps with high poundage + 3 sets of 20 reps with light poundage.
(this suggestion for already-fit tyro).
Weight gaining = THE SQUAT above all other exercises. Alternate squat with straight arm pullover (see CHEST): i.e. do 1 set of 20 reps with squat; then 1 set of 10 reps with pullover straight off; then rest a minute; then another set of 20 reps with squat; then another set of 10 reps with pullover straight off; then more rest; etc., etc., etc. Total should = 3 sets of 20 reps for squat; 3 sets of 10 reps for pullover. (Note: other weight gaining exercises in this programme can = deadlift/curl/bentover rowing/bench press/press behind neck. ALL q.v.)

Making squats easier . . .

(a) Always warm up first to = muscles supple/elastic.

(b) Keep skull up especially when coming UP for better balance.

(c) Note: coming down to HALF squat will only stress *thigh* muscle rather than BACK as well. Going down all the way gives you the works.

(d) Ramrod back straight to focus work on thighs in this instance (rather than hips/lowerback).

(e) Use wood block/paperback/thick book under heels for stability.

(f) Pile on gradual/even/smooth squat rate. Avoid quick collapse and resulting bounceup effort. Harmful.

(g) Concentrate/concentrate/concentrate ON doing perfect SQUATS. Once mind wanders you've had it.

Memo: SQUATS = basis of BIG legs + BIG chest/shoulders/POWer.

IMAGINE squat weights glass-sided safes crammed with 7,500 silver dollars weighing 1,300 lbs. to hoist and YOURS if YOU do it (has been done).

Solo leg extensions

As shown.

Strap old iron/books/dumbells (or proper iron boots) weighing enough to give you stick. On feetsoles.

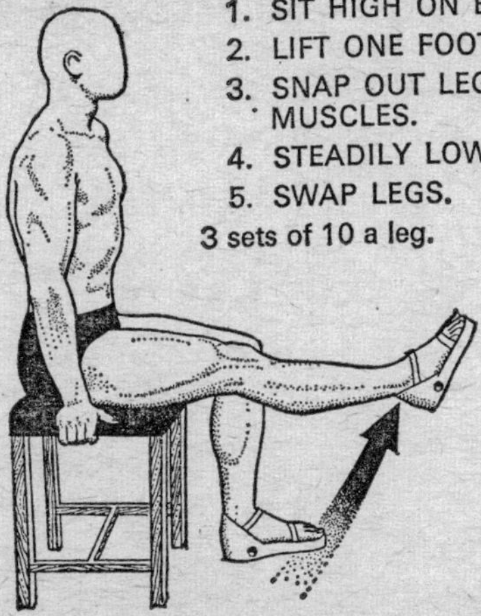

1. SIT HIGH ON BENCH/CHAIR/STOOL.
2. LIFT ONE FOOT FROM FLOOR.
3. SNAP OUT LEG TENSING THIGH MUSCLES.
4. STEADILY LOWER LEG TO START.
5. SWAP LEGS.

3 sets of 10 a leg.

Leg curl

1. STAND STRAIGHT PUSHING ON WALL.
2. VIGOROUSLY FLEX KNEE RAISING KNEE HIGHEST BEHIND YOU.

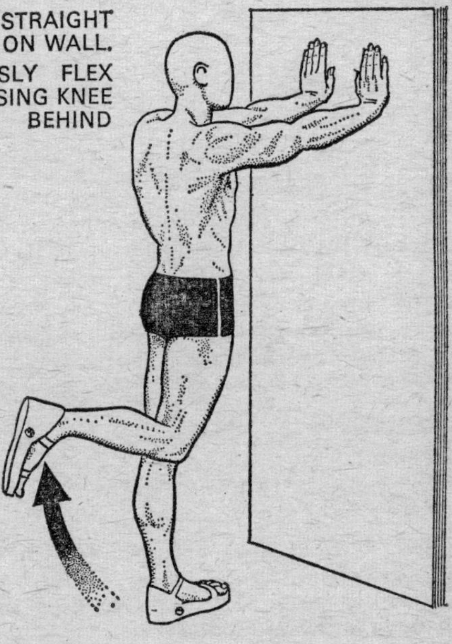

3. TRY TO BEND KNEE JUST A BIT MORE EACH TIME.
4. FEEL THIGH BICEPS BURN.

Note: massage thighbacks immediately if cramp-prone.

2 sets of 10 a leg.

OR do *Thigh Curl* with mate's help

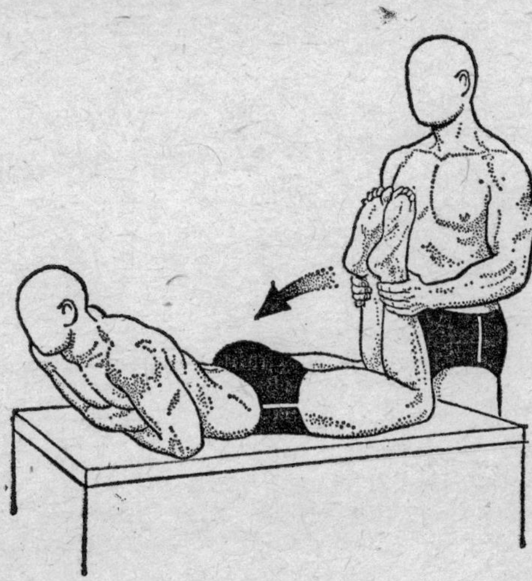

1. LIE FLAT ON TRAINING BENCH.*
2. SHOVE LEGS OVER EDGE.
3. TRY/TRY/TRY TO CURL LEGS TO GLUTES WHILE...
4. MATE HAULS BACK HEELS.

2 sets of 10.

Note: partner MUST not resist too much so that you lock solid.

**=make training bench from plank 6 ft. long 18 in. wide, covered with blanket. And jack it up on bricks/books/boxes.*

Straddle lift

As shown.

1. STRADDLE BARBELL GRIPPING BOWS/STERN.
2. RISE ERECT.
3. LOWER BODY BENDING KNEES FOR 15 in.
4. COME BACK UPRIGHT.

Note: keep back STRAIGHT and YOU too can hoist heavy weights with this thigh booster.

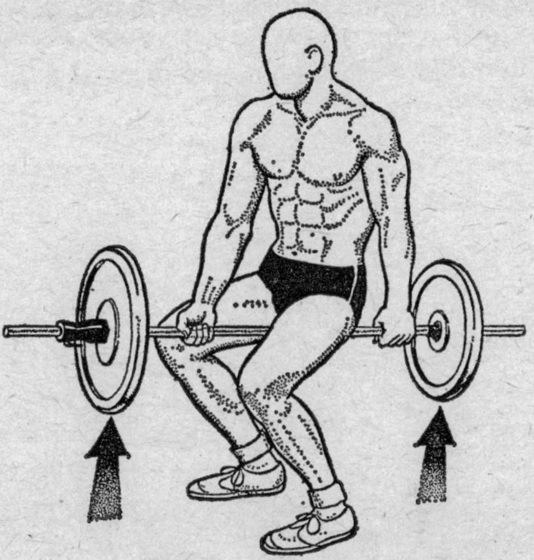

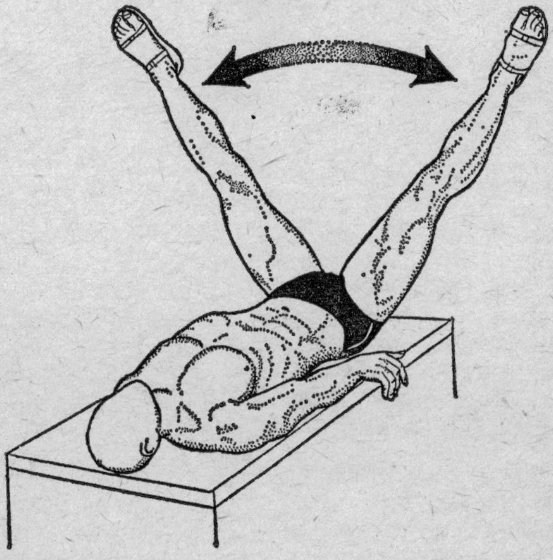

Leg splits
As shown (booted-up)

1. LIE DOWN.

2. RAISE LEGS AT 90 DEGREES TO TORSO.
3. SUBMIT LEGS SIDEWAYS INTO SPLIT POSITION.
4. BRING TOGETHER AND LOWER.

Note: press on floor with flat of hands.

Also . . .

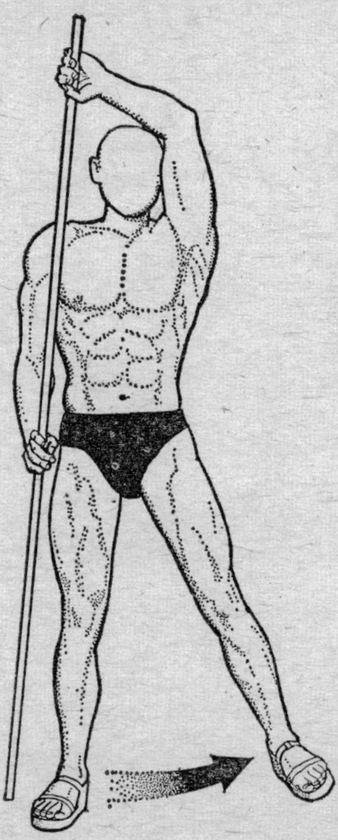

1. GRIP VERTICAL DOOR JAMB/POLE/ROD.
2. RAISE WEIGHTED RIGHT LEG SIDEWAYS.
3. LOWER AND REPEAT.

Then swap legs. 2 sets of 8 reps.

Hack squat

As shown.

1. PROP HEELS ON 2 in. WOOD BLOCK WITH BARBELL BEHIND ON FLOOR.
2. CROUCH AND GRASP BAR.

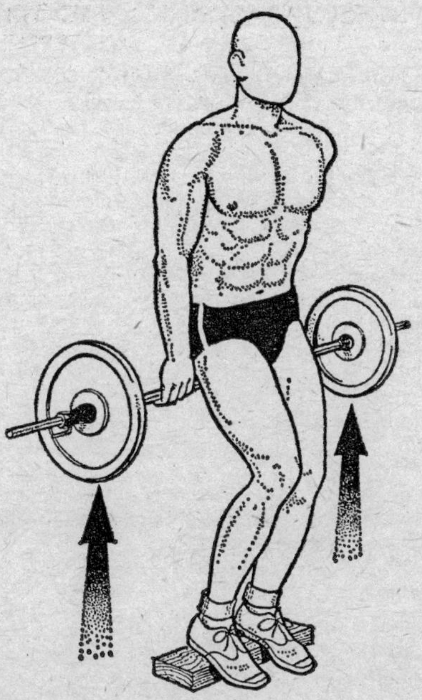

3. SHOVE/SHOVE/SHOVE WITH LEGS UNTIL...
4. BAR RUBS THIGHBACK.
5. STAND STRAIGHT.
6. LOWER AND REPEAT REPS.

4 sets of 8.

Front squat

1. REST BAR ON DELTS (SHOULDERS) FROM THE FRONT.*
2. CARRY OUT SAME AS ORTHODOX SQUAT...
3. BREATHING IN ON THE DOWN; OUT ON THE UP.
4. AND RESTING HEELS ON 2 in. BLOCK.

**= secret: clean bar to shoulders (see BACK); raise elbows high in front; let bar roll down palms to slightly hooked fingers; bar should rest across delts IF elbows are lifted and grip is just over shoulder width.*

Note: use lighter poundage. And only use this as variant on normal SQUAT (after first two 6–8 weekly sessions).

POWER PLAN FOR GASTROS

The calves.

NEVER forget these (though easy to). GO/GO/GO for big/strong/bulging lower legs with enthusiasm. They need HARD graft (miles from heart + tissuebuilding blood food No. 1 queue spot).

Work calves hard to equate them with showman's traps/pecs/fists. Massive chest/tiny calves look ridiculous. NEVER hurry/rush/skimp calf work as token gesture. Calves WILL grow if you concentrate.

Tapemeasure thickest calf part after lifting foot off deck and pointing toes. Ankle measurement = thinnest part just above jutting bone.

Note: ALWAYS work calf muscles through FULL movement range. Go to very top on tiptoe AND thrust heel right down on return. If cramp . . . massage by jamming thumbs deep into calf belly and working in circular motion. Carry out for 2 minutes after training.

Heel raises

As previous. BUT with loaded barbell across shoulders. Use 3 in. wood block etc. 30 reps.

Donkey raises

As shown (place wood block 2–3 feet in front of stool).

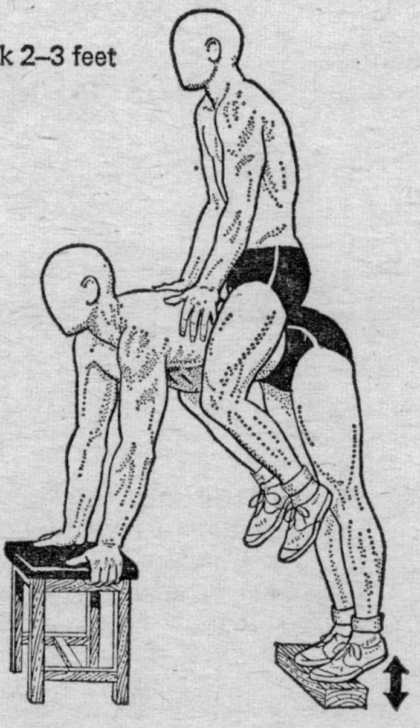

1. STAND TOES ON BLOCK.
2. BEND OVER AND GRAB STOOL TWOFISTED.
3. MATE SITS ON BACK LIKE DONKEY-RIDING.
4. LOWER/RAISE HEELS.

30 reps. Work up to 4 sets of 15.

Sitting calf raise

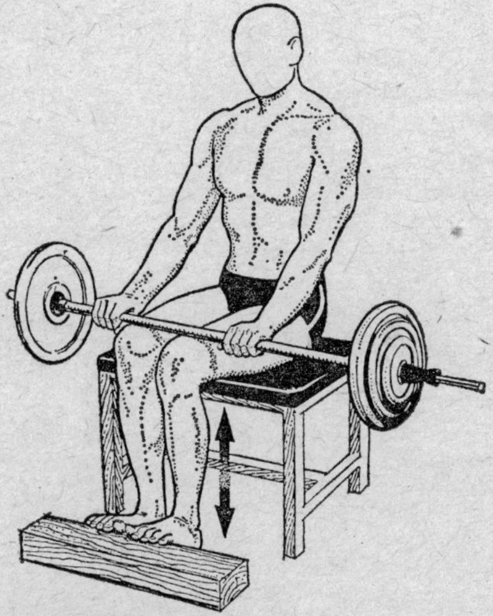

(YOU can take a lot of weight here).

1. CHAIR SIT, BARBELL ACROSS KNEES.
2. REST TOES ON 2–3 in. WOOD PLANK/BLOCK/BOX.
3. LIFT HEELS HIGHEST YOU CAN . . .
4. TENSING GASTROS HARD/HARD/HARD.

3 sets of 15.

Straddle jumping

1. HOLD BARBELL ACROSS SHOULDERS.
2. JUMP UPWARDS . . .
3. LANDING ON TOES, FEET ASTRIDE AND . . .
4. IMMEDIATELY LEAP BACK UP . . .
5. LANDING ON TOES FEET TOGETHER.

Note: spring from FOOT ACTION ALONE (hardly bending

knees). Really it = feet astride jumping with barbell. Pad neck-back.

Calf walking
Grasp heavy barbell across shoulders. Walk around WITH exaggerated heel-toe action. Finally—walk tiptoe for 2 minutes. Maximum = 3 minutes.

Toe raisers

1. STAND HEELS ON 3 in. BLOCK, BARBELLS ACROSS SHOULDERS.
2. LIFT FEETBALLS OFF FLOOR.
3. ROCK BACK ON HEELS AND...
4. RAISE TOES UPWARDS.
5. LOWER/REPEAT.

3 reps of 15.

Single calf raise
As shown.

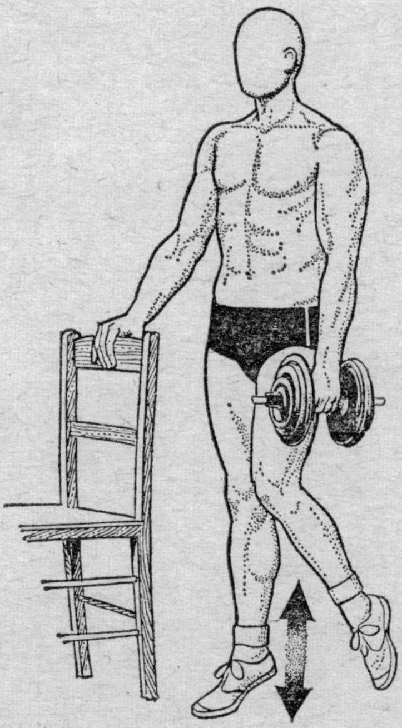

1. GRIP HEAVY DUMBELL IN ONE HAND...

2. CHAIR BACK WITH OTHER.
3. RAISE ONE FOOT OFF FLOOR.
4. DO SINGLE CALF RAISE WITH OTHER ON EXTREME TIPTOE
5. LOWER AND REPEAT.

2 sets of 10 a leg.

ABDOMEN

ABDOMEN: 4

YOUR ABDOMEN should be a muscular wonderwall as flat as a handslap. And which, with a deep breath OUT plus HARD tensing, should weather into a chiselled column as rugged as Alpine granite.

SHOULD, yes. But DOES it? Are YOUR abs showing YOU up as a bad insurance risk (a paunch *does*)? Is YOUR pot belly pregnant with prolapsis/hernia potential; YOUR waist carrying baby power instead of manly strength?

Paunches 15 per cent bigger than chests = expectancy of life chopped by a quarter. Let MR TOUGH keep YOU out of the coffin by trowelling abs, shaving waist, reviving liver/bowels/etc., with gutpowering diet and exercise.

WHAT YOUR ABS CAN DO TO-DAY

IF you scored at least "average" in guts-test (see BODY). If NOT see abdominal care (below); *and* skip these for moment.

Breathe from stomach

Do daily as *excellent* toner.

Blow out all lungair and drag stomach in furthest possible. Count up to 8 then relax stomach wall again. Keep repeating (in car/bed/office) aş TONIC for abs wall/midriff/alimentary canal.

Isolate recti

Press hands on thighs and CONTRACT in spectacular central forward isolation the 2 recti muscles of the abs. Blow out lungair first. Then drag abs right back. Then (with practice) contract prominent recti muscles for 6 seconds. Holding breath.

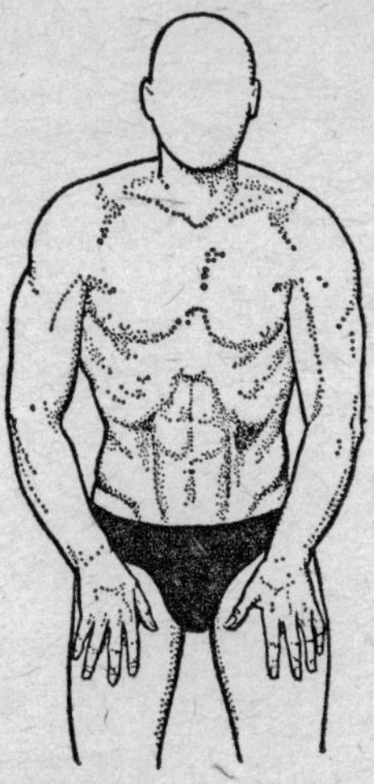

SEE TO YOUR ABS/WAIST TO-DAY

Before taking ANY exercise.

Slim down first

IF overweight with gutprow DO NOT TRY ANY situp or toe touching toners from standing. Slim down first to = bending without discomfort. Or danger.

Eat properly

Vital for trim midsection.

WORSHIP high protein diet which = MUSCLE.

ABHOR big carbohydrates/fats intake (*some* needed for energy/chemical balance/etc. BUT excess of either = body fat).

GANNET *smaller* meals more frequently to keep body ALWAYS nourished. And waistline slim.

SCRAP junk foods from factories (in tins/boxes/packs). Sweets. Artificial carbohydrates (chips/pizza/etc.). Hot dogs. Salami. Egg noodles. Ice cream.

WOLF *really* NATURAL FOOD (REAL MEAT/REAL MILK/REAL EGGS).

MUNCH cardboard box as well as breakfast cereals (about as much natural nourishment in contents).

NOSH w-i-d-e-s-t range of GOOD wholesome food to = a

balanced diet. ALL kinds of meat/fish/seafood. And whole grain cereals. Poultry. Fresh fruits. Greenest greens. Both raw/cooked. Use shotgun method hitting out with wide food choice so *much* of it will do YOU good.

MISS OUT on white sugar (and all its products). Skip pies/cakes/ cookies. And doughnuts. Pastries. Candy bars. The lot.

Note: refined sugar robs body of vitamins which YOU need to make MUSCLE. Gives you quick energy shot for 2 minutes; that's all. STICK to natural sugars (as in vegetables/fruits/ wholegrains).

DIAL-A-DIET using milk shake-type bodybuilding supplements containing ALL food nutrients in right amounts (especially proteins/vitamins). Supplement chews too. See muscle mag ads.

DAILY WAIST TONING

Take YOUR pick. Or skip altogether IF flat-abbed NOW. And roaring fit.

Memo: so much depends on what YOU want and CAN do (on age/build/urge).

Leg lift

As shown.

Lie on back. Lift legs high together. Lower slowly. Best results = when lowering them to 6 in. above floor and holding (counting

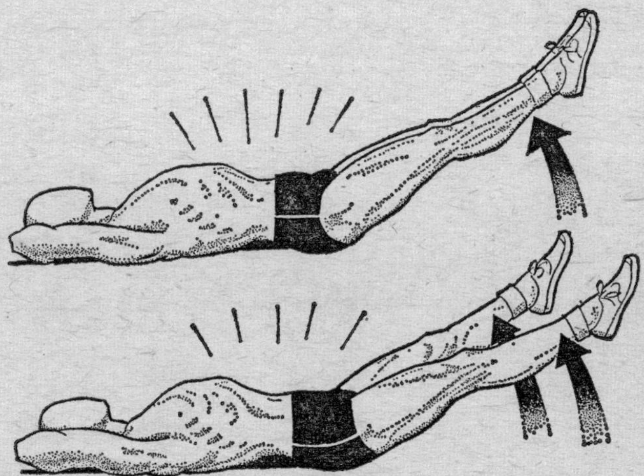

→

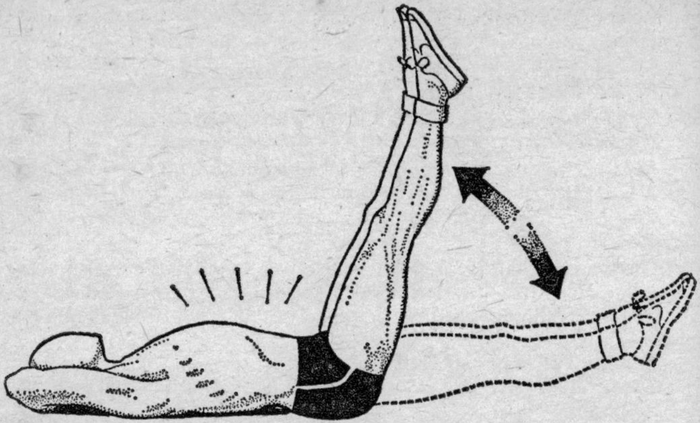

to 10). Extra best = spreading legs during the count then joining them before dropping to floor.

10 reps maximum at first. Work up to 15 slowly. And lengthen holding-count to 15–20.

Note: at first cheat by bending knees if you find HARD work. Give exercise all you have.

Reverse bridge

As shown.

HARD exercise.

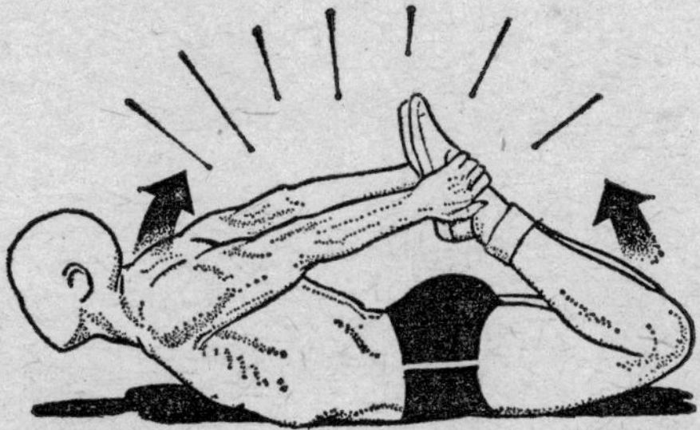

Lie prone on floor. Bring hands back to grip legs. Arch back/pull arms. And raise chest/thighs off ground. Tyros limit: 5 reps.

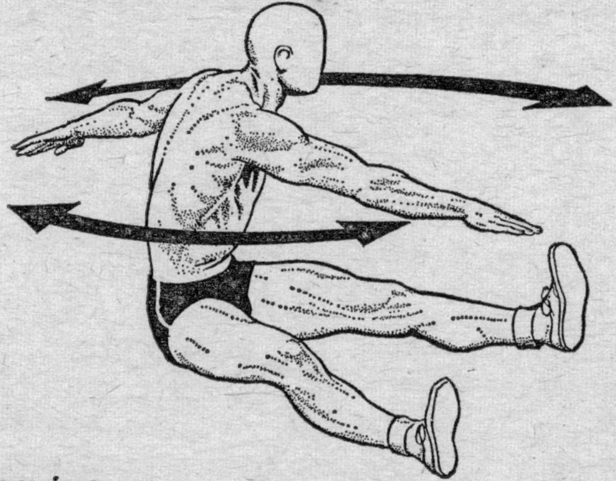

Toe swings

As shown.

Have legs flat on floor. Keep knees straight (though cheat at first). IF toe-touching not possible at first it soon will be (few sessions makes YOU looser).
(See also BACK.)

Push ups

Keep heels flat down, straighten legs/arms. Push glutes high. Bend arms. Lower body near floor. Push back to glutes-in-air position (arms/legs straight). NOW keep arms FULLY extended and lower bottom half of body to floor.

Work up to 20–30 reps.
(See also ARMS/CHEST/BACK/LEGS.)

Bath legup

As shown.

Raise legs alternately and together (more water in bath = easier it is).

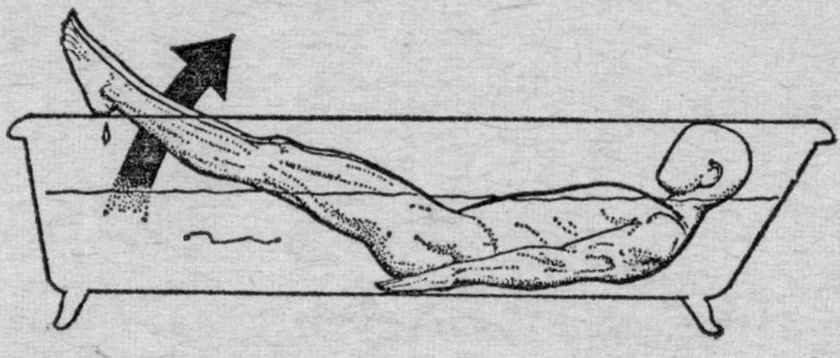

Then contract into small ball.

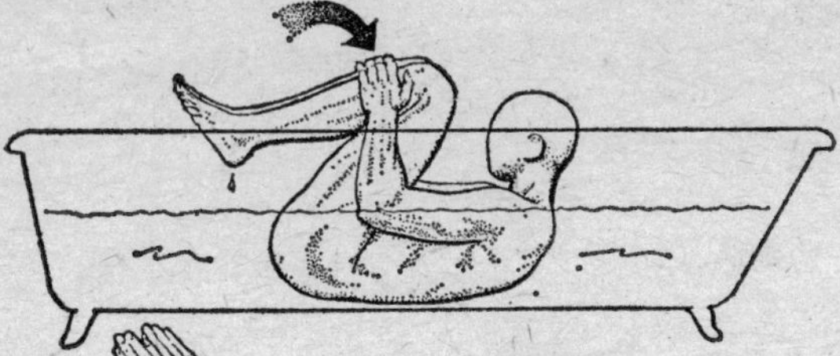

TV toners

As shown.

Try these in chair, position by position. Try bending arms in second position.

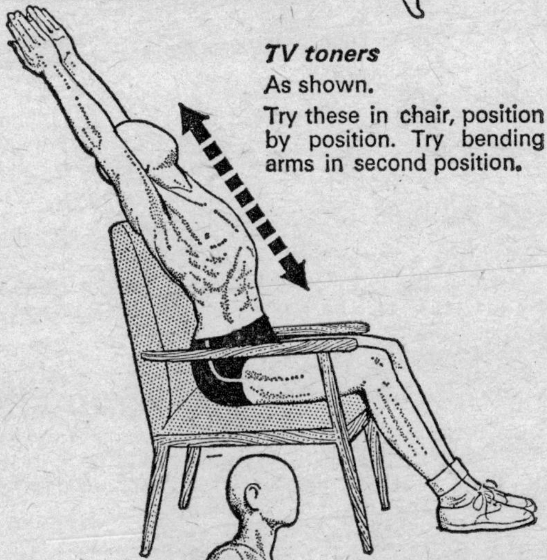

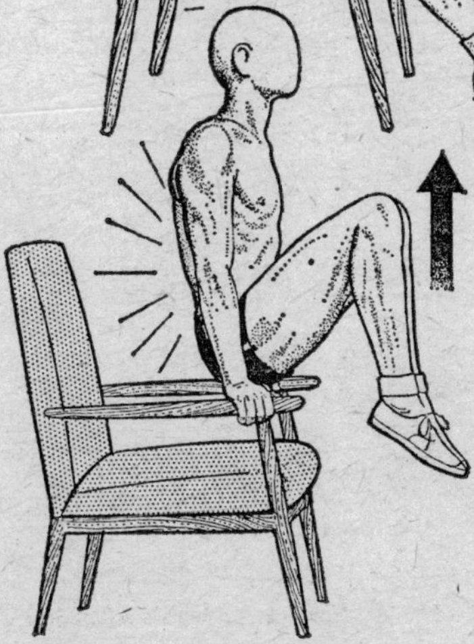

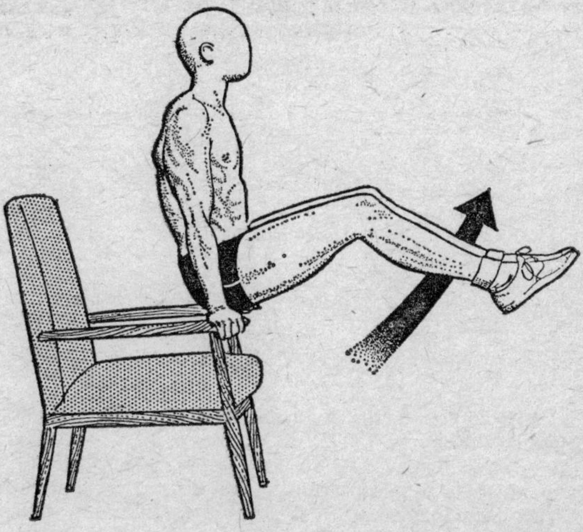

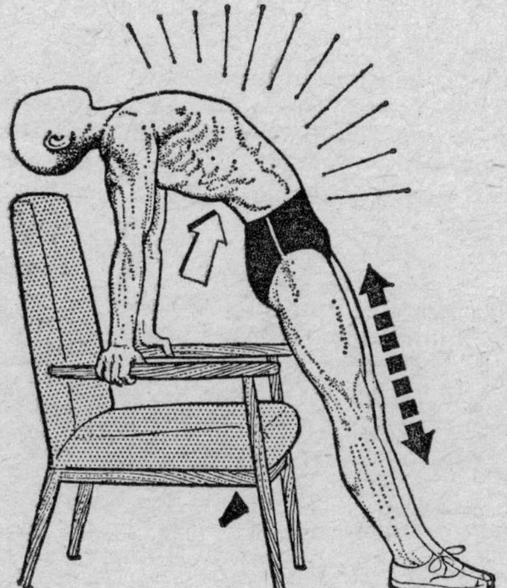

Situps

As shown.

Lie on floor looking up. Stretch arms behind head. Have feet trapped under furniture. Take deep breath and sit up blowing out. Now lower trunk to floor (breathing in).

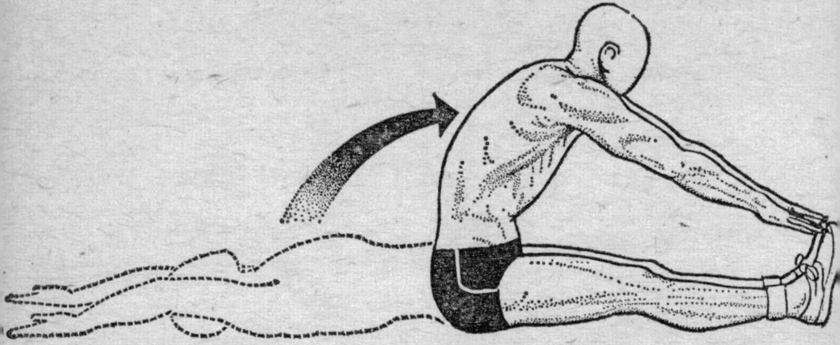

3 sets of 20 reps make solid/flat/hard gut. Slimmers need 40 FAST reps. Potbellied must NOT do this at all if overweight and find it strainful. Those over 45 need fewer reps: 3 sets of 10 for flatgut; up to 20 reps for reducing will do.

NEVER overdo situps. Rest 3 minutes between sets when feeling workout effects.

Note: light book held behind head adds resistance as YOU progress to stronger stomach.

Situp variant

Lie flat on back feet hooked under heavy object. Mesh fingers behind neck. At count of ONE take normal breath in and slowly sit up (chin tucked down). Try to touch elbows to knees. At TWO count lower body to floor exhaling. 25 reps = fine progress.

Legup variant

Lie flat on back legs outstretched. Press hands on floor or clasp at headback. At count of ONE take breath-in and slowly lift legs to point up at ceiling. At TWO-count slowly lower legs from vertical to floor exhaling as you do. Aim = 25 reps.

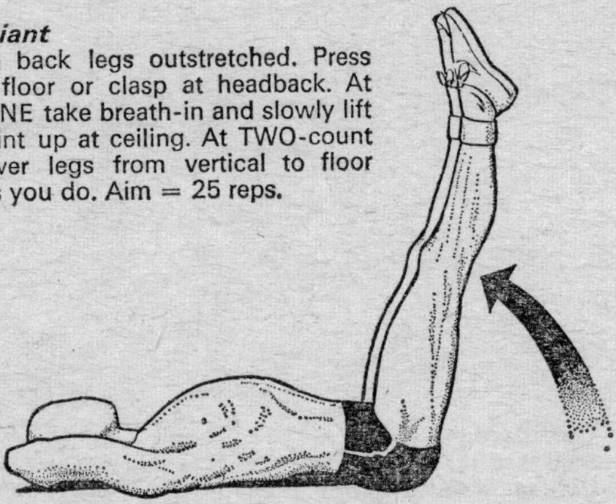

INSTANT MINIPOWER FOR WAIST

Situp spoiler
Lie on floor kneesup holding book behind head. TRY to sit up pulling with ALL strength against gravity. For 6 secs. Note: if already tough enough to raise torso use heavier book so attempts frustrated.

Lower abs contraction
Lie looking up hands clasped behind neck or at sides. Deep breathe in. Raise and hold legs to 14 in. height . . . for 6 seconds.

Upper abs contraction
As above BUT . . .

Clasp hands behind neck and RAISE torso 15 in. off floor: 6 seconds. Expect difficulty at first.

Cobra
Lie prone/legs together/palms resting by chest (fingers forward). Take deep breath. Lift head/trunk up and back at same time as straightening arms. When arms fully stretched toss back head (hold 6 seconds).

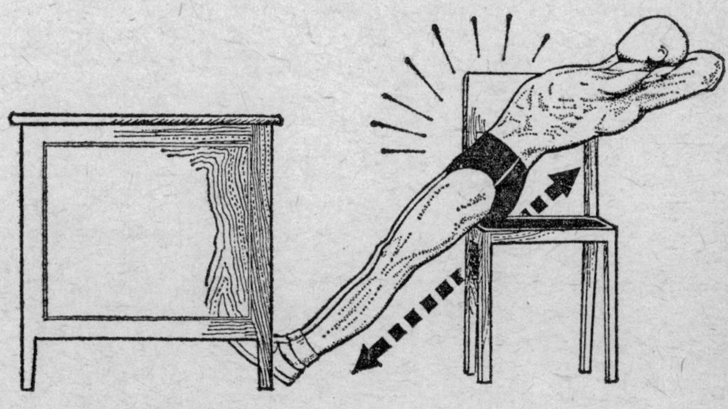

Desk toning
Trap toes under desk while sitting. Hands behind head. Go right back (as shown) for 6 seconds.

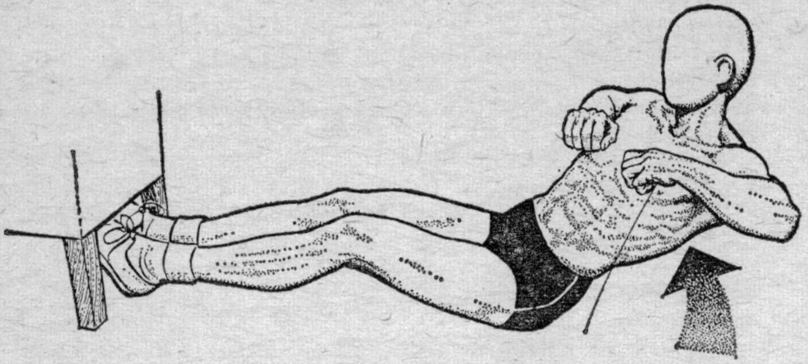

Situp check

As shown.

Trap feet secure. Hold in this situp position 6 seconds.

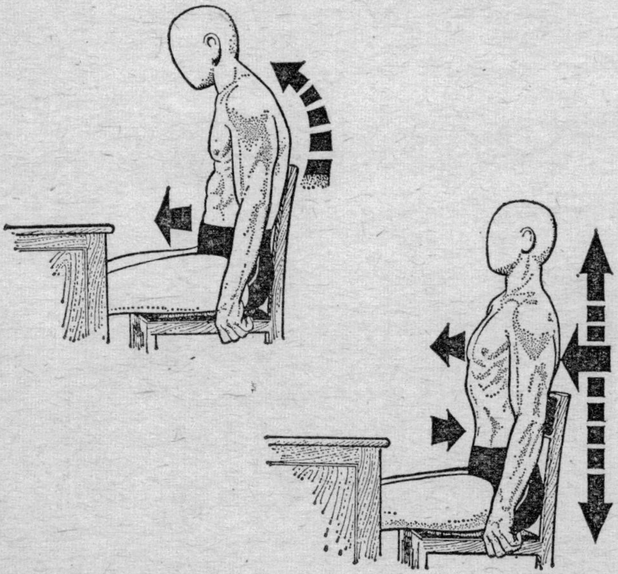

Stomach tensioner

As shown.

Let guts flop. Retract stomach muscles by contraction (NOT breathing in). Hold hard for 6 seconds breathing normally.

ABDOMEN WAIST POWER PACKING

Tapemeasure waist across navel when standing (chest normally lifted): don't try to drag in abdomen. Best test = pants-slipping-down-rate.

Tapemeasure hips across centre of glutes when contracted (NOT relaxed).

Champs use abdominal board to ironout midriff. Muscle mag ads show good ones. BUT 6 ft. plank about 18 in. wide will do at first (covered by blanket or foam rubber). Tilt at all angles as necessary using furniture etc.

Just a few sets on this board and POWer. Those abs/obliques = relief map of strength.

Remember:

FOR general fitness + stamina = 3 sets of 20 reps on any one or two of below exercises.

FOR weight gaining (IF now underweight) = NOT much abs work at moment. 2/3 sets of leg raises or situps ample (too much abs work keeps weight down).

FOR reducing weight = 3 sets of 2 or 3 different abs exercises (20/30 reps).

FOR abs POWer = sets of 10 reps with heavier resistance.

DANGERS: watch boredom risk (waist training needs few *weights* exercises as body weight often enough resistance; also reps usually high). Make up for any interest that weights would add *by getting stuck in*. And give those abs some stick.

Choose that MON/WED/FRI, etc., routine from. . . .

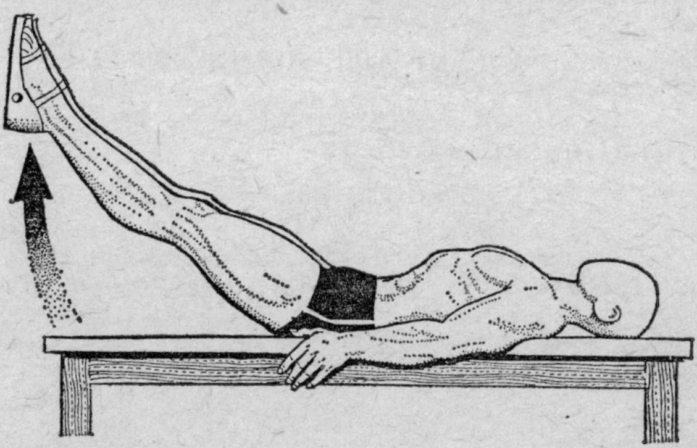

Leg raise

Have bench level as shown.

Lie on bench (or on floor). Raise legs upwards until feet touch bench/floor behind head. Progress to wearing iron boots/dumbells/any old weight strapped to feet.

2 or 3 sets of 10 reps.

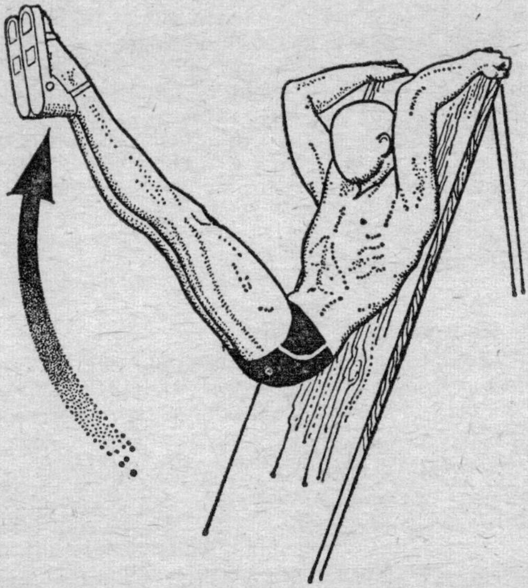

On inclined board

As shown (with plank slanted at 40 degrees).

1. LIE ON BOARD HEAD AT TOP.
2. REACH UP AND GRIP TOP TO STOP SLEDGING DOWN.
3. RAISE LEGS HIGHEST THEY GO (BREATHING OUT).
4. PAUSE BRIEFLY THEN ...
5. LOWER TO STARTING POSITION.

2 or 3 sets of 10 reps.

Note: As abs *really* toughenup YOU will be able to lift hips off plank after legs already raised. Makes it even better abs power-packer.

YOU have 2 ways of adding resistance for progress. Slant board steeper OR wear iron boots.

Situps

As shown.

As done earlier (with arms stretched behind or at neckback). Can be done on abs board with feet locked under a strap at end. When YOU can do 25 reps (head coming over knees) YOU can progress to inclining board.

Slant to 40 degrees. Lie ankles under strap. Clasp hands behind neck. TRY to touch brow to knees. Steadily unroll to starting position.

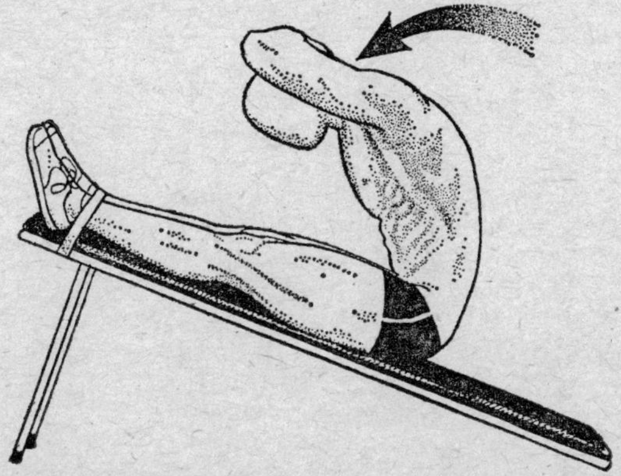

Memo: breathe out as you go up, in on coming down. Keep back rounded (to power abs instead of stressing on thigh strength).

2 or 3 sets of 10.

Progressive resistance = slanting board steeper. Or by adding weight with barbell held at back of neck (as shown).

Alternate kick

Don iron boots/dumbells/books strapped to feet.

Lie on floor looking up hands behind head. Draw alternate legs back to abs then LASH each limb forward (lower to floor slowly after each rep).

When you become REALLY tough keep feet clearoff ground ALL the time. But NEVER in early stages.

2 sets of 15 reps rythmically.

Sidebend with dumbell

As shown overleaf.

1. STAND FEET ASTRIDE WITH 20 lbs. DUMBELL IN LEFT HAND.
2. BEND BODY TO FURTHEST RIGHT...
3. LETTING RIGHT HAND SLIDE DOWN RIGHT THIGH.
4. RETURN TO VERTICAL.
5. DO SAME REPS NO. FOR OTHER SIDE TOO SWAPPING DUMBELL.

30 reps with dumbell in right hand, 30 in left.

Note: DO bend sideways NOT forwards. Come back up straight

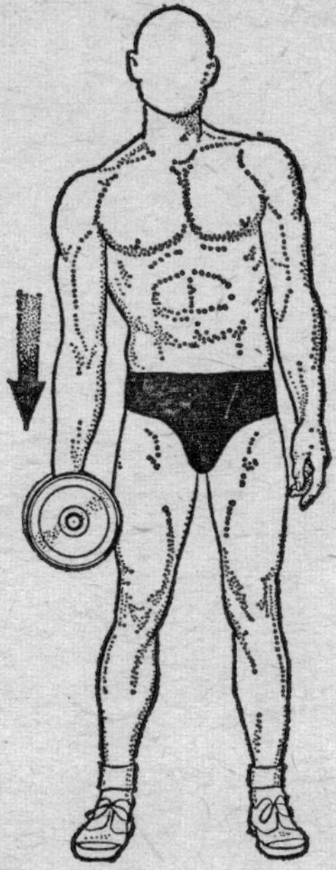

each time. Can be done bending body both ways each time as far as possible left and right.

Barbell sidebends
As shown opposite.

1. STAND FEET APART BARBELL ACROSS SHOULDERS.
2. BEND BODY BOTH WAYS FROM SIDE TO SIDE...
3. AS FAR AS SPINE ALLOWS.

Note: ensure barbell collars locked so weight discs secure.

Trunk twisting
Start with barbell held as above.
Now rotate trunk first right then left.

Kneesbent situps
As shown opposite.

1. TRAP FEET UNDER BARBELL (OR ABS BOARD STRAP).
2. MOVE UP TORSO SO KNEES BENT AND CLASP HANDS AT NECKBACK.

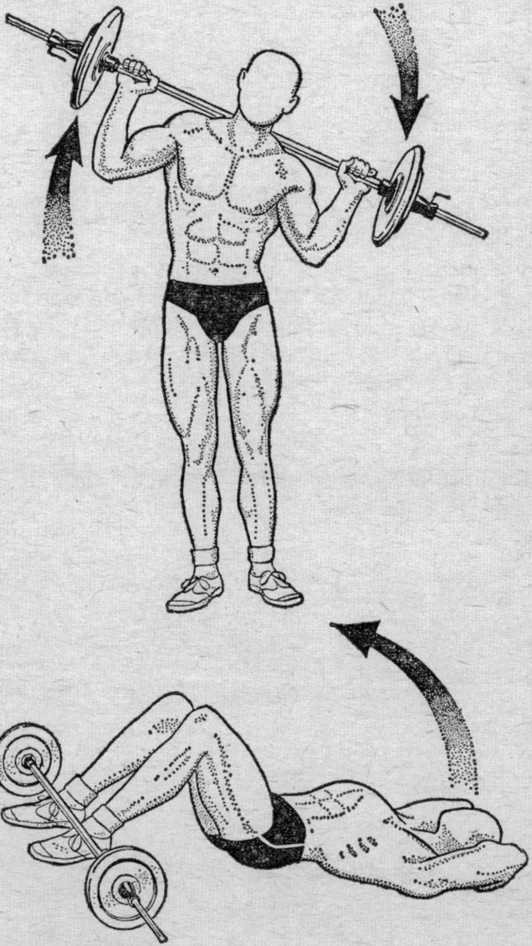

3. SIT UP BY . . .
4. ROUNDING THE BACK BIT BY BIT UNTIL . . .
5. HEAD COMES WELL OVER KNEES.
6. UNROLL SMOOTHLY TO START.

3 sets of 10 reps.
Note: breathe out as YOU sit up.

Twisting situps

Lie on level abs board, feet under strap. Hands clasped behind head. Start to situp BUT this time twist torso so right elbow brushes left knee. Return to lieback position. Do other side next same way: touching left elbow to right knee.

A winner when done on inclined board.

Continental roll

1. STRAP ON IRON BOOTS AND LIE DOWN ...
2. KNEES FULLY BENT/HANDS TO SIDE/FEET DRAWN WELL UP.
3. LIFT FEET OFF FLOOR, THEN HIPS, THEN ...
4. ROLL OVER TO TOUCH SHOULDERS WITH KNEES.
5. REVERSE MOVEMENT LOWERING FEET TO FLOOR.

Note: keep legs fully bent right to the end. As YOU toughenup ⇒ do it on inclined board for peak power.

Sandbag situps

As shown.

Hold bag at necknape. Hook toes under chair etc., when weight upsets balance.

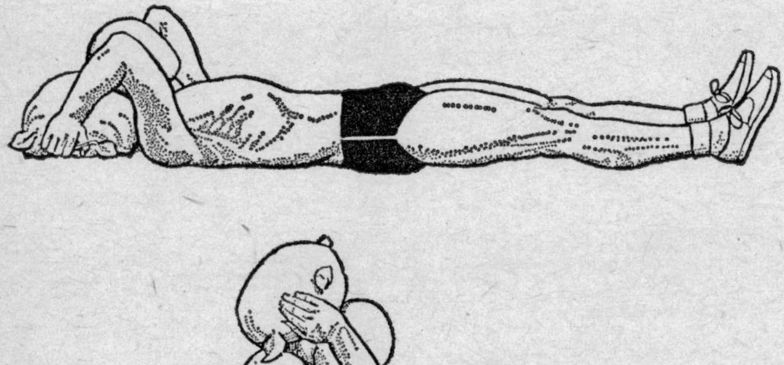

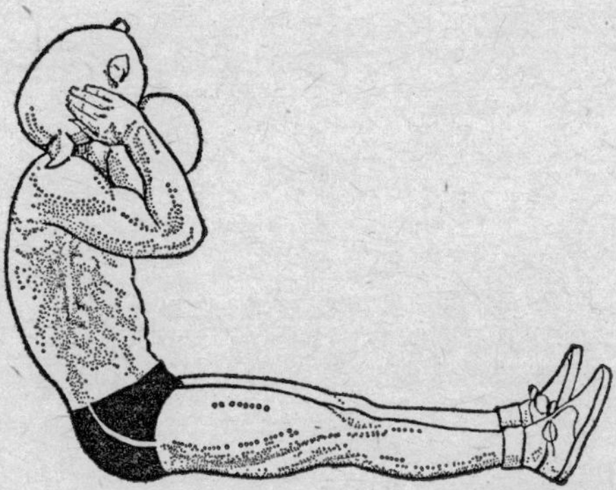

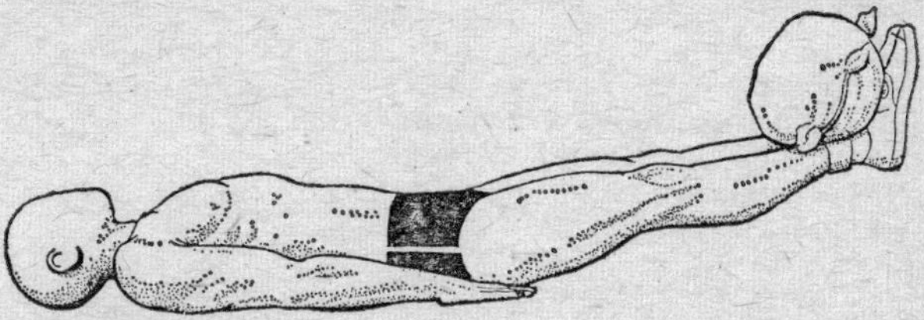

Sandbag leglifts

As shown.

With sandbag on shins. HARD exercise for building hard/hard/ hard abs.

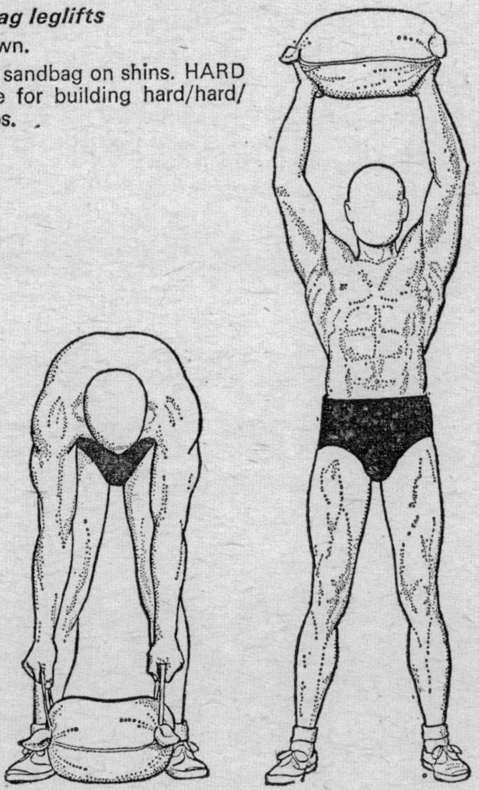

Sandbag snatch

As shown.

Grab sandbag off floor and up overhead in ONE smooth motion. Practice rythmic movement.

CHEST/SHOULDERS/BACK

CHEST/SHOULDERS/BACK: 5

MODEL THE TORSO of YOUR dreams with razorsharp exercise/hammering effort/fretsawing enthusiasm to = glassfibre muscle-fibre. Chopoff fat here, chipin bulk there (add MUSCLE everywhere). Look on gluetube chest/celluloid shoulders/balsawood back as YOUR own kit of bits. And toolup with MR TOUGH. However: different kits = different models. Temper that dream towards the possible model you can *become* on what YOU have going for you to-day. To-morrow you may be heading for a MR OLYMPIA build from skinny/fat beginnings (there are always exceptions). BUT be realistic for the moment.

Usually . . .

OXFAM AD CONDITION =
= MANLY/FIT/ERECT TORSO KIT.

MICHELIN MAN BUILD =
= SLIM/TOUGH/TAUT TORSO KIT.

BOY WONDER PHYSIQUE =
= MR UNIVERSE-AIM TORSO KIT.

Draw up YOUR torso plan to-day. And give it ALL your ALL.

CHEST

YOUR CHEST is a powerhouse. Throbbing with heart/lung power, pulsing with vital arteries/veins, buttressing vulnerable vertebrae/organs, here is THE heartland of crushing power potential. Yet it could be in terrible shape. Start by stretching/mobilizing your rib cage THEN buildingup those pecs (arm muscles sited on chest). Benefits = MANLY appeal; BIGGER lungs; VIRILE posture; SURVIVAL against injury; SELF confidence; INTEREST in powergrowth (chest readily responds to effort). Not ALL will reach 50 in. Herculean chest. But go as far as YOU can.

WHAT CHEST WILL DO TO-DAY

Give YOU encouragement.

Grow quickly

Using HARD resistance = quickest gains. Quite normal to add 2 in. to chest (expanded) within 14 days of iron-throwing. Even 1 in. growth after ONE session with weights IS possible. Note: boom due to extra chest mobility (does NOT carry on at this rate).

Shows endurance reservoir level

Try test for 15–60 year olds.

1. BEND DOWN WHILE CHAIR-SITTING SO ...
2. HEAD IS BETWEEN KNEES.
3. BREATHE IN MOSTEST SITTING UP.
4. HOLD BREATH FOR ...
5. AS LONG AS POSSIBLE.

Score =

+70 seconds = REALLY fit.
50 seconds = Average fit.
—30 seconds = Doctor check.

Blowup hot water bottle

Some can burst this thickrubber balloon.

Try various shapes/sizes. Go for fairly perished one. Practise

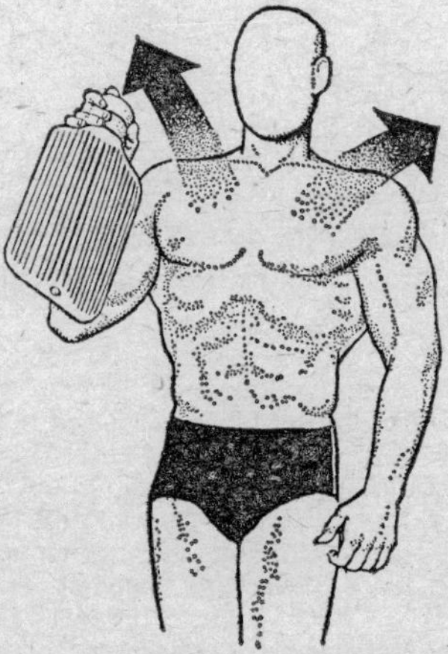

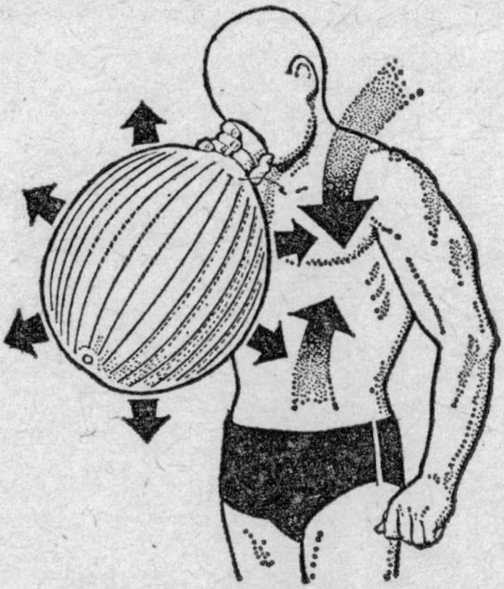

deep breathing (see later). Brace first. Grip neck very firmly (so no blowback). Put mouth to hole/cup with hands/give breath-blast.
Warning: go easy AT FIRST. YOU can go dizzy (and flake out). Balloon rubber in easy stages.

Beat breathalyser

Expect HARD blowing-effort.

As bag is being put together . . .

1. BREATHE IN/OUT QUICKLY AND QUIETLY.
2. WHEN TOLD TO FILL THE BAG . . .
3. COUGH (RIDDING MOST LUNGAIR).
4. TAKE HUGE BREATH OF AIR DRAWN-IN QUIETLY.
5. FILL THE BAG NONSTOP.

THIS = more chance of passing test than any other. Reason: THE fresh/clean/new air being jetted into breathalyser from YOUR just-exercised lungs.

Make nonswimmer stay afloat

As shown overleaf.

1. KEEP FACE DOWN/LUNGS FULL OF AIR/BODY VERTICAL AND . . .
2. HEADBACK JUST ABOVE WATER (ARMS/LEGS DANGLING).
3. KEEPING HEAD HORIZONTAL RAISE FOREARMS TO BROW AND . . .

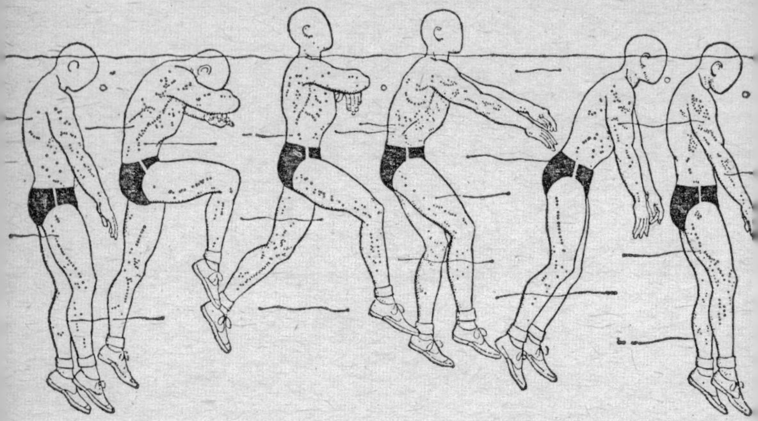

4. ALSO ONE KNEE ALMOST TO CHEST WHILE OTHER FOOT IS STRAIGHT AND RAISED BEHIND.
5. NOW LIFT CHIN TO REST ON WATER AND BREATHE-OUT THROUGH NOSE.
6. SWEEP ARMS OUTWARDS/DOWNWARDS SLOWLY AND SCISSORS KICK FEET TOGETHER (BREATHING IN THROUGH MOUTH).
7. NOW LOWER HEAD AGAIN.*
8. BACK TO ORIGINAL REST POSITION.

*=*IF sinking PUSH down with extended handpalms.*
Note: keep repeating cycle NEVER holding breath until gasping for air.

CHEST CARE

Clamp mouth shut in fogs/smoke/fumes. In lorry-slowed car cut off airflo vents. In industrial smuts close down car heater. Go crazy gulping fresh air WHEN you find it. Go walking/camping/beachcombing. ALWAYS make most of FRESH air.

DO avoid fresh air fanatic image.

Remember: regular deep breathing habit = automatic reviver makes you less susceptible to oncoming fatigue.

Ease a stitch

Stitch is spasm of the diaphragm. Most common cause—eating just before taking violent exercise. Easiest way of avoiding, don't eat large meals before violent exercise. For relief of symptoms, bend down five or six times touching toes, decrease rate of physical exercise.

Check a pain

Pain in chest can mean nothing or something. Any athlete who is unfit, in the process of getting fit will have some pain and discomfort in the muscles of the chest wall, as he is vigorously using unused muscles. This must be distinguished from pains caused by heart disease, and stomach pains which occur in the gap between the ribs.

Chest pain related to the heart commonly occurs between the ages of 45 and 65; presents as gripping pain round the chest, particularly in the centre of the chest, sometimes radiating down the left arm.

Stomach pains usually in pit of stomach just above umbilicus, usually associated with meals, and possibly the bringing up or down of wind (flatulence).

If in doubt of any chest pain related to exercise, particularly if over 40, seek medical advice.

DAILY CHEST EXPANDERS

Vest best chestpacked through HARD resistance exercises. BUT daily chest limberers best first for unfit/old/young.

Experiment with all. Choose routine. Stick/stick/stick at it.

Deep breathing

As shown overleaf.

Stand straight with hands loosely by side. DEEP breath in. Slowly raise hands forward. And up to over head position (keeping arms straight). Feel ribs bellowing out to utmost as you S-T-R-E-T-C-H up/up/up.

Breath should blend WITH movement (both ending same second). Pause for a second. Lower arms to side breathing out.

Keep body UPRIGHT. Don't overdo it at first (dizzy spells = you ARE).

10 reps a day initially. Increase by 1 every 2 days.

Post-exercise unwinders

ALL good for unravelling tension AFTER powerpacking session. They give better chest mobility.

(a) Lie looking up on floor, arms sideways, palms flat on floor. Lift chest off floor, breathing in slowly on lift. Breathing out on lower. 12 reps.

(b) Stand feet astride, arms forward, fingers pointed. Part arms slowly bringing shoulderblades back. Return to start breathing hard out.

(c) Stand astride, hands on lowerhips. Breathe in slowly through nose (feeling ribsflare and slight abdomen distension at start). Lift head slightly back. Breathe out slowly. 12 reps.

(d) Stand astride. Circle arms forwards/upwards to brush

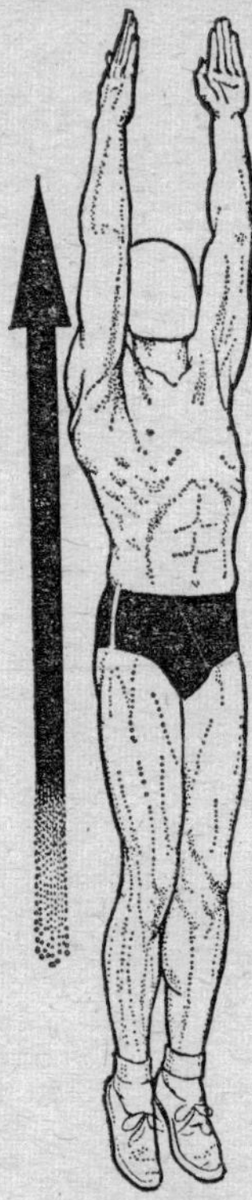

Deep breathing

ears. Then slowly down. Swing a total circle with both arms. Breathe in slowly through nose on upward arc and out on downward one. Stretch fingers. 12–15 reps.

Chest stretch

(See also LEGS.)

Do straight after deep knee bends (WHILE breathing heavily).

1. REST HANDS AT SHOULDER WIDTH ON MANTEL-PIECE, ETC.
2. KEEP LEGS STRAIGHT/BODY RIGID/BACK A BIT INCLINED.
3. BREATHE IN DEEPLY, BLOWOUT CHEST TO LIMIT AND . . .

4. PRESS DOWN HARD BOTH-HANDED.
5. RELAX/REPEAT.

10 reps working to 20. And bigger rib cage.

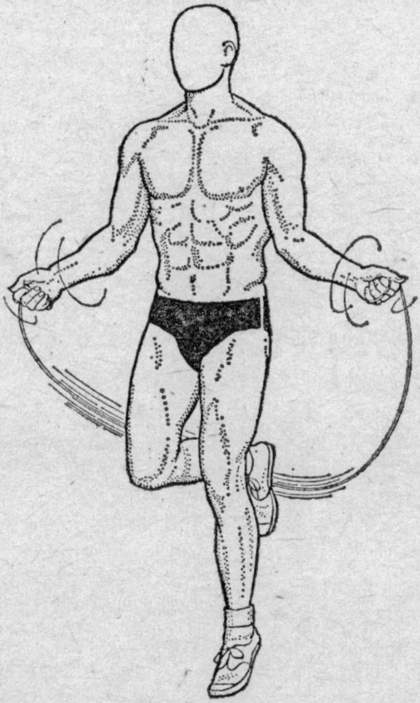

Rope skipping
1 jump per rev. 2 jumps per rev. Alternately 1 *then* 2 jumps per rev.

Pumper
As shown.

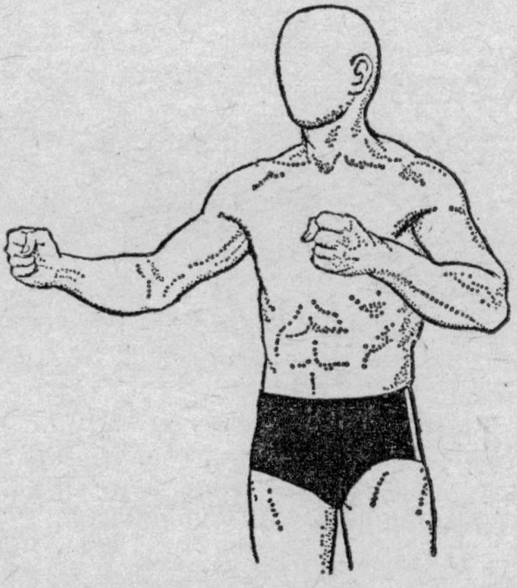

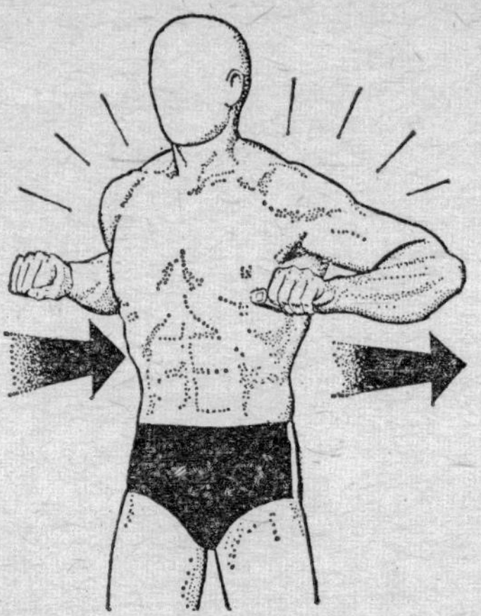

Extend arms to front. Hands open or clenched. Snap elbows back to furthest point. Inhale as arms piston back; exhale as limbs shoot forward. 25–30 reps.
Note: snapback = REAL cheststretch value.

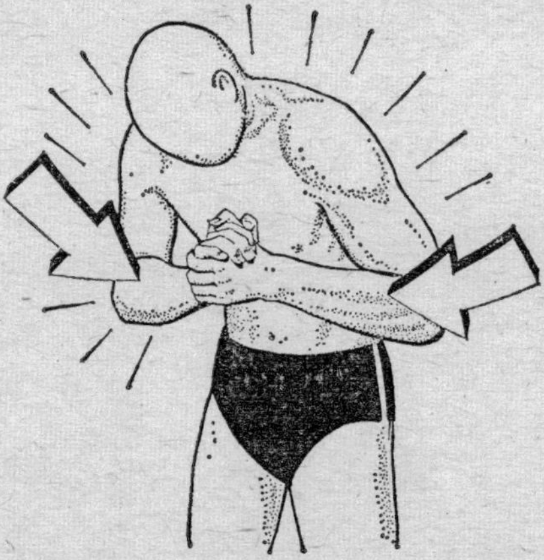

Clasper
Clasp hands palm to palm in front of chest. Press like mad in jerking actions. FORCE must come from UPPER arms (*not* lower). Feel pecs contract (to buildup muscle).

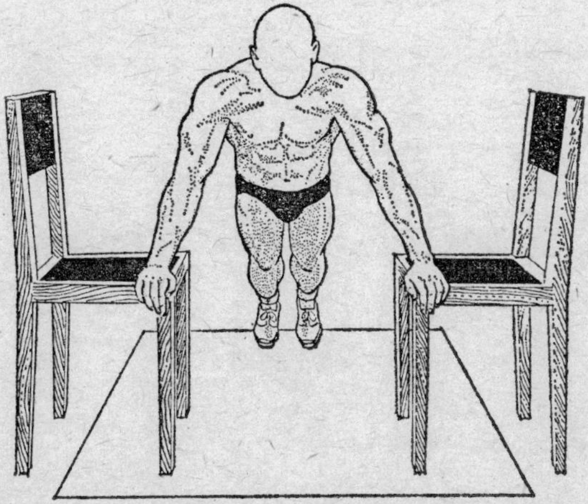

Dipper
Place 2 chairs as shown. At shoulder-width. Go up/down.

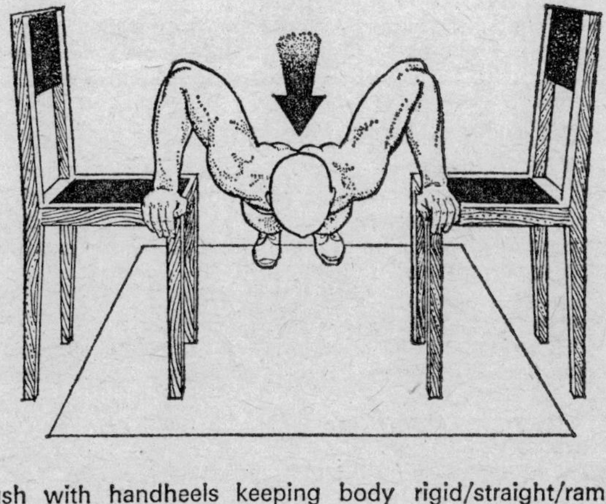

Push with handheels keeping body rigid/straight/ramrod. Do 10 reps each session first 14 days. Slowly go to 25 reps. HARDER than normal pushups.

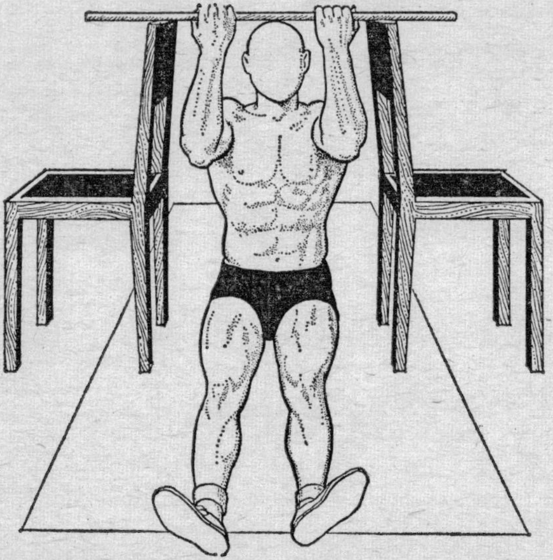

Chair chinner
Place broom handle across 2 chair tops (ensure they won't tip). Sit between. Pull on bar. Chin to it. Hold body straight, resting

---

INSTANT CHEST MICROPOWERS

Seated thigh press
Sit legs apart. Feet flat on floor. Handpalms on outside of thigh muscles (midway between glutes-kneecaps). Back straight. Breathe in and press HARD (6 seconds). Spread thighs outwards o battle hand pressure.

Bent-arm hands press-in
Clasp hands at chestfront. Raise elbows horizontal. Upper/lower arms should = 90 degrees. PRESS hands for 6 seconds together.

Hands press-in straightarmed
As above.
BUT with arms straight out in highdive position. 6.

Bent arm press-overhead
Bend arms clasping hands directly overhead so elbow joints

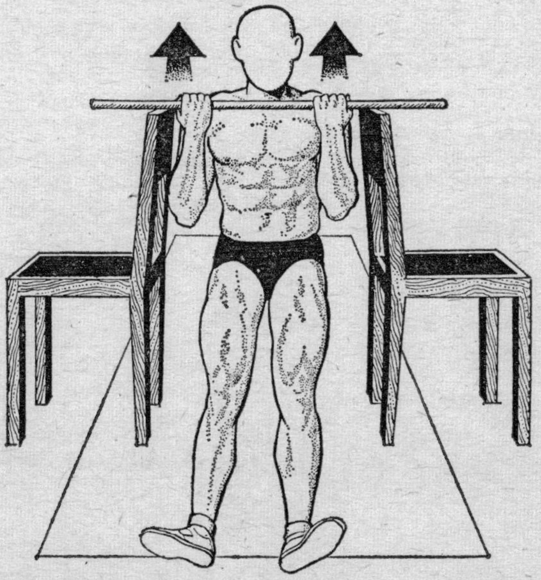

on heels: THE advanced aim. In the beginning just do chinups from sitting posture.

---

make 90 degrees corners. Keep elbows out at sides. Stand straight. PRESS hands for 6.

Wall thwarter
Stand 18 in. from wall. Spread arms sideways straight. Press palms on wall and, bracing with legs, PUSH both-armed as though TRYING to arc hands together through wall. 6 seconds.

Door baulker
Stand in doorway facing jamb. Place chestlevel hands on each wall sandwiching jamb (handheels towards body/elbows bent out/forearms floor parallel). Breathe in and VICE jamb for 6.

Squeeze-in gripper
Sit/stand. Handsgrip bucket/kettle/basin sides 4 in. from chest (so elbows at 90 degrees). Take deep breath. TRY to crush object in 6 second collision.

Lateral raise
Lie on floor with arms full stretched to side level with shoulders (palms up). Place 2 table chairs so each handheel can press under each chair seat. Weight these down with books. Try to jackup chairs keeping arms straight. 6 seconds.

Straight arm pullover
Lie full length on back this time with weighted chair behind head. Reach out palms under seat (under 20 in. from floor). Get ready with arms shoulder width apart and PUSH up. 6 seconds, arms *straight.*

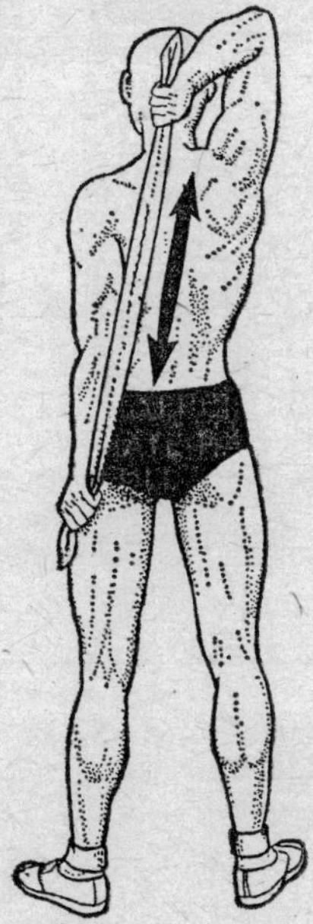

Arm extension with towel
As shown (from behind head).

Get into position. Take towel in wide grip in body front, pull taut with stiff arms, swing overhead in wide arc. Lower left arm until straight down by left side (fist in by upper thigh; knuckles front). Hold. TRY to force right hand up overhead. 6 seconds fight.

PILING ON CHEST POWER

Open throttle slowly. CHEST thrives on harder and harder graft. Swing changes in chest exercises as much as possible over

6–8 week sessions. ALL powerpacking variants should be used at one time or another.

Truly mighty chest does NOT come from massive armour plating of chest muscle. It starts from full/high/deep rib box. Attack this first with: deep breathing toners; hi-rep squats which = *deep* breathing; pullover exercises.

NEVER use massive weights. Just enough to make you concentrate on every rep with the last 2 a REAL tussle to complete.

Bench press = No. 1. CHEST builder (basis of ALL chest routines). Squats (alternating with pullovers) excellent. Add 2 sets of bent arm pullovers/floor dips/flying. Inclined bench movement = good for a change.

POWER PACKING FOR CHEST

Attack rib cage weaknesses first. THEN nailon muscle armour-plating.

Tapemeasure blownup chest across nipples (arms to sides). Fully inflate/tense chest/ramrod back. Best test = when shirt buttons fly off with chest normal.

Breathing squat

With heavy barbell on shoulders. (See also LEGS.)

1. STAND FEET 12 in. APART TAKING 3 FULL BREATHS.
2. HOLD LAST BREATH, BEND KNEES, SINK TO SQUAT AND . . .
3. RETURN UPRIGHT BLOWING OUT.
4. DO 3 MORE BIG BREATHS . . .
5. AND CARRY ON.

3–4 sets of 12–15 reps will make YOU gasp (and blowup rib box).

Note: keep back straight; raise heels on 2 in. wood block.

Follow with . . .

Barbell pullovers

As shown.

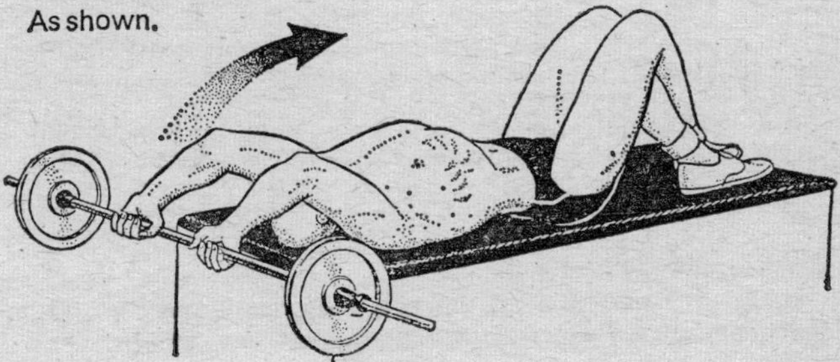

1. LIE ON BENCH OR FLOOR.
2. DRAW KNEES UP AND CROSS LOWER LEGS.
3. GRASP BARBELL SO HANDS SPACED 12 in. APART, ELBOWS SLIGHTLY BENT.
4. LET BARBELL TRAVEL BACK OVERHEAD AND START TO . . .
5. INHALE WHEN BAR DIRECTLY OVER EYES.
6. KEEP INHALING UNTIL BAR REACHES LOWEST POINT BEHIND HEAD.
7. SWING BACK UPWARDS TO OVER-EYES POSITION AND . . .
8. HOLD BREATH UNTIL HANDS OVER FACE AGAIN.
9. BREATHING OUT COMPLETES MOVEMENT.

IF using bench keep feet on IT (*not* floor). Knees *up* ⇒ relaxed abs + MORE room for rib box expansion.

3–4 sets of 10 reps.

Note: Super Sets system with squats (and barbell pullovers). Use 3–4 sets of squats at 20 reps each *with* sets of pullovers. Thus: do set of squats; THEN set of pullovers; THEN rest; THEN set of squats; THEN set of pullovers; THEN a second rest; etc., etc. Until all sets finished. Can be done with other exercises (e.g. bench press *and* flying).

Parallel dips

(See also ARMS.) *see diagram opposite.*

1. HAVE HANDS/ELBOWS SPACED WIDE APART.
2. CHIN ON CHEST/ROUNDED BACK/FEET UNDER FACE.
3. RELAX ABS TOTALLY AND . . .
4. AS YOU START TO LOWER BODY RIGHT DOWH INHALE SO YOU GET FULL LUNGFULL AT DIP BOTTOM.

Warning: be patient/careful with this rib box expander. You are NOT going HERE for ace triceps (see ARMS again). Do NOT arch back/pullback elbows/breath once. Instead: do double bounce (or stretch) at dip bottom AND simultaneously take short breaths SO you feel rib cage flareout as air pumps to lungs bottom.

TRY to relax rib box as you do exercise. Be patient. NEVER rush. Waist weight to add resistance NOT needed if dips done OK.

Dumbell pullover

Similar to barbell technique.

Bring up knees. BUT if difficulty balancing plant feet over bench end on to floor. *see diagram opposite.*

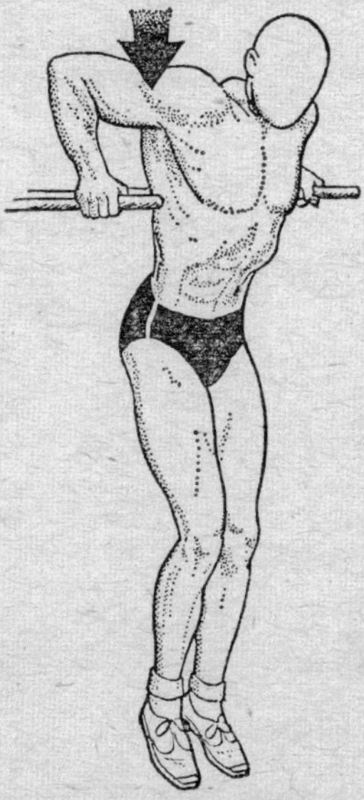

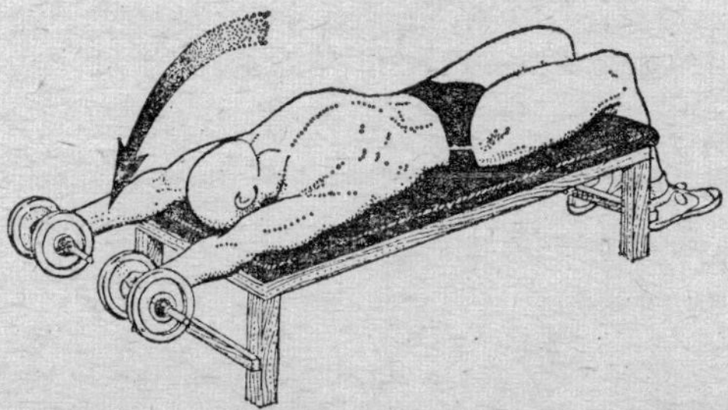

1. HOLD DUMBELLS WITH STRAIGHT ARMS OVER CHEST (KNUCKLES TO REAR).
2. STEADILY LOWER ARMS BACK TO WAY BEHIND HEAD.
3. DROP THEM FURTHEST POSSIBLE BEHIND (INHALING).
4. BLOWOUT AS ARMS GO BACK TO START.

3–4 sets of 10.

AND *now for pecs bombardment to = bulletproof muscle plates on* CHEST.

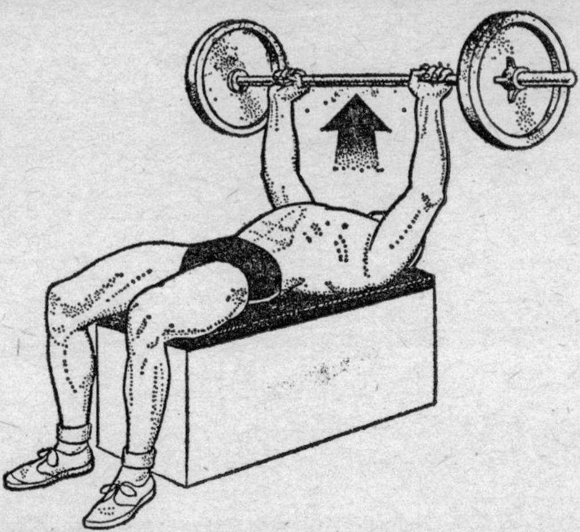

Bench press
VITAL powerpacker.
As shown.

1. LIE ON EXERCISE BENCH.
2. HAVE MATE HAND YOU BARBELL OVER CHEST AT YOUR FULL ARMS' STRETCH.
3. INHALE AS YOU LOWER BAR TO CHEST AND ...
4. EXHALE AS YOU PUSH BACK.
5. GIVE IT STICK.

3–4 sets of 12–15.

TERRIFIC single movement for *torso* in same league as squats. And deadlifts (see BACK). Low reps = POWer; high reps = stamina; medium reps = weightgainer.

Dumbell bench press
As above (save weights differ).

Unless using very heavy weights no need for mate to hand you dumbells. *Don't* have palms facing here.

Sets of 5–6 reps = POWer; 8–12 = general bodybuilding; 15–20 = stamina.

Flyers flat
As shown.

Similar start to dumbells bench press BUT as bells are lowered they fly AWAY from body.

1. GRIP DUMBELLS WITH STRAIGHT ARMS OVER CHEST (PALMS FACING).
2. BEND ARMS AND CARRYAWAY FROM TORSO INHALING AND TURNING ...

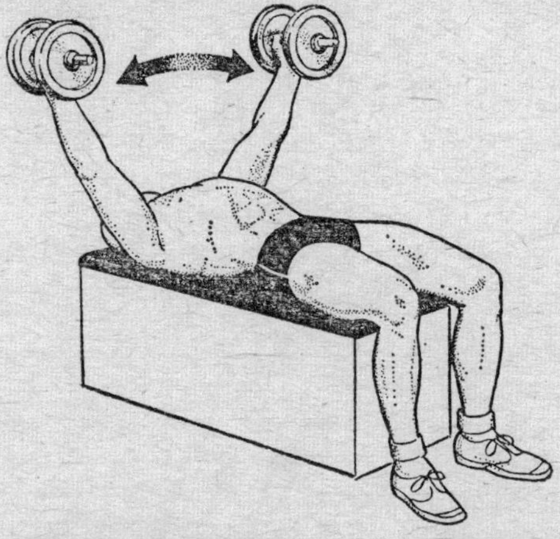

3. FISTS OUTWARDS AS BELLS ARE LOWERED (FORE-ARMS VERTICAL).
4. EXHALE AS YOU PRESS BACK STRONGLY TO START OVER CHEST.

3 sets of 12 reps. Use light poundages so YOU cope.

Flyers decline
As shown.

Same as above BUT on inclined bench (good for SHOULDERS too). Use 40 degrees slant.

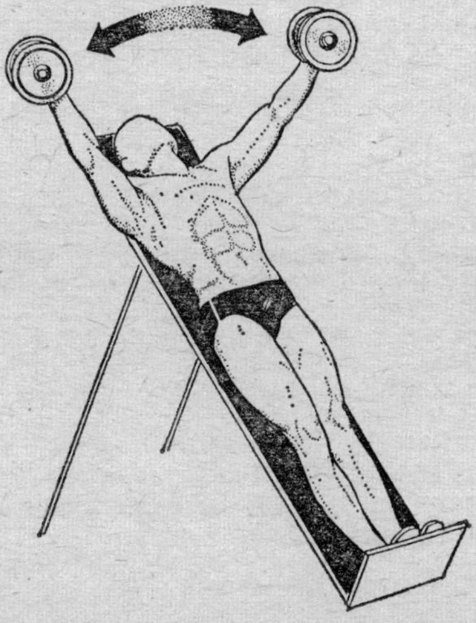

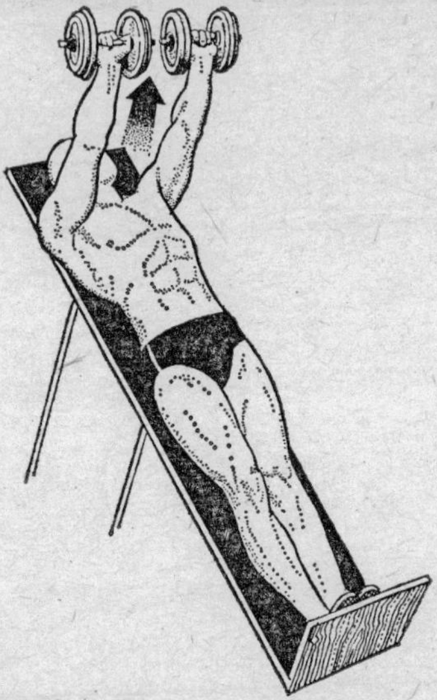

Incline dumbells bench press
Like bench press with bells (save for 40 degrees slanting board). Just lower bells to shoulders NOT away from body as in flying.
Use all weights YOU can handle for 3 sets of 10 reps.

Floor dips
Pushups with feet on box. Inhale as torso is lowered, exhale on UP. Later add weight on back to add resistance (book say).
8–12 reps = general strength; 15–20 reps = stamina. And one with rubber inner tube . . .
STRETCH tube in front of AND across chest (as shown opposite).

SHOULDERS

BUNCHED SHOULDERS punch fists/saltwater/balls NOW. Pack YOURS with rocketbig force (NOT pocketmini power). Stitch a REAL shoulderpadding of 3-way musclecladding (front/side/back) into this wet suit, that T-shirt, these denims. And throw away cardboard suits as YOUR deltoids start to swell with thickness and shape from soaking them in workout sweat. ALLangle exercise tailoring makes a torsotop the hallmark of manhood. Have MR TOUGH as YOUR tailor and cut a REAL dash.

WHAT SHOULDERS CAN DO THIS MINUTE

Give vital help to ALL torso/arm POWer (see also FINGERS/HANDS/WRISTS).

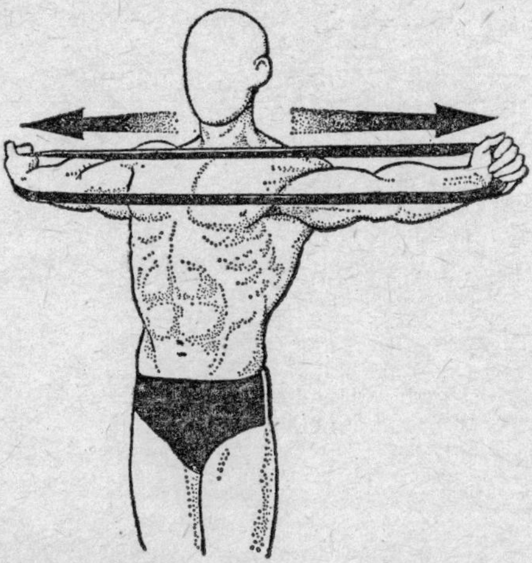

Ease carrying loads
(See also LEGS/BACK.)
Lifting ends with swinging object on to shoulder. Balance with 1 hand as you walk. Swap sides en route to skip strain.

Boost pushing POWer
As shown.
(See also LEGS/BACK.)

1. BEND BOTH LEGS AND JOCKEY SHOULDER AGAINST OBJECT.
2. BEND ARMS COMPLETELY BUT GRIP WITH HANDS SO THAT . . .
3. OBJECT SHIFTS FORWARD (AND UPWARD AT YOUR END) AS YOU STRAIGHTEN LEGS WITH POWERPUSH.

Note: useful for crate-like objects which need edge lifting to swivel/slide into position. AND *shoulders* take THE weight.

Support 15-stone man
Small man perched (BUT braced) on rockface footholds can be plinth for BIG man mountaineer reaching high handholds over granite bulge (Victorian climbers' cheating method).
Situation is . . .

1. YOU ARE PROPERLY BELAYED TO ROCKSPIKE WITH NYLON ROPE (AND HAVING EXPERIENCED CLIMBING MATE) AND . . .
2. NEED TO SCALE BLANK 8 ft. ROCKWALL SO YOU . . .

3. CLASP HANDS NEAR CRUTCH AND LEAN ON ROCKFACE.
4. MATE STEPS ONEFOOTED INTO YOUR HANDGRIP USING YOUR HEAD AS HANDGRIP FOR BALANCE.
5. THEN HE STEPS UP WITH OTHER FOOT ON TO SHOULDER.

And reaches handholds above.
Note: REAL mountain stuff this (like handjam in FINGERS/HANDS/WRISTS). Shows delts' toughness needed to jackup big boots + man's weight.

Broom-lift with shoulder POWer
(See also FINGERS/HANDS/WRISTS.)
Lift broom off floor by grasping handle *end*. Hoist with straight-arm strength. To shoulder height.

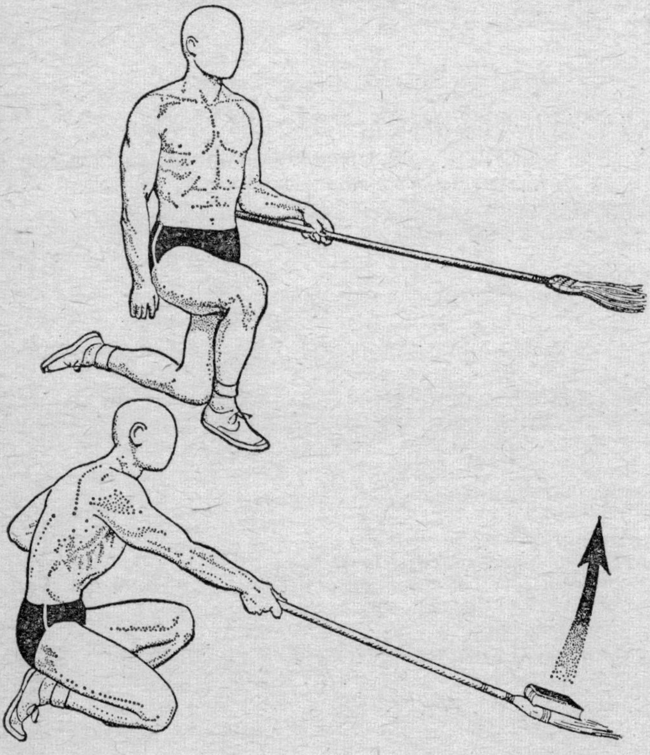

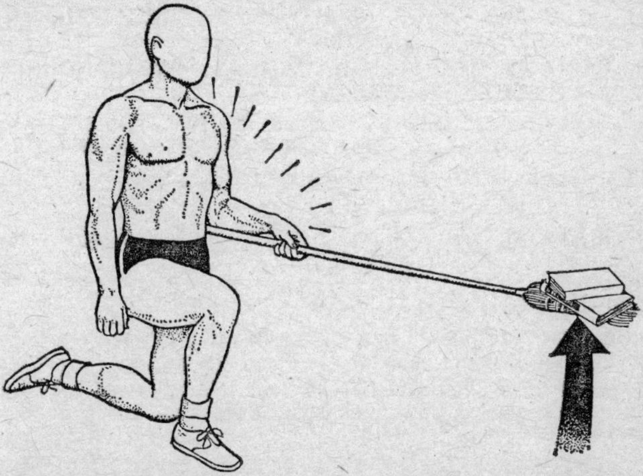

Practice with elbow bent at first (holding towards broom end). Work lifting grip towards far end of broom handle until YOU can do this feat. Straightarm lift will beat most of YOUR friends.
THEN practice with extra resistance (book on broom top) for real POWer test.

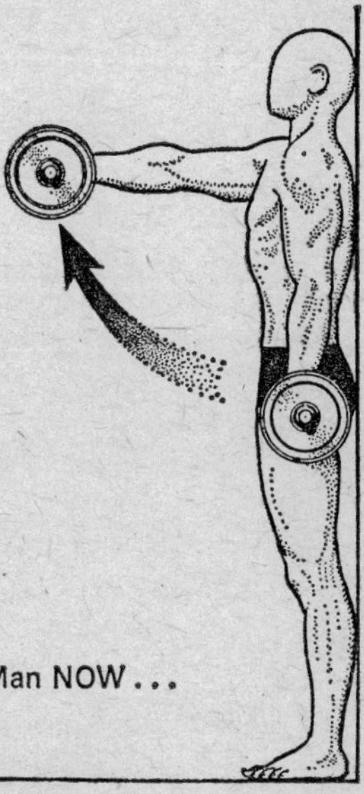

Hold heavy weight to front
ACID test of STRENGTH.
If YOU fancy chances as Strong Man NOW . . .

1. STAND PRESSING ALL BACK TO WALL (HEELS/GLUTES/SHOULDERS).
2. GRIP DUMBELL (OR WEIGHT LIKE SANDFILLED KETTLE) IN ONE HAND.
3. KEEPING ELBOW STRAIGHT TRY TO RAISE IT STRAIGHT TO FRONT AT SHOULDER LEVEL.
4. HOLD FOR 60 SECONDS AND ...
5. LOWER STEADILY/SLOWLY.

IF *you* can hold fully loaded dumbell for minute YOU really have TREMENDOUS strength.

DAILY SHOULDER TONERS

(See also ARMS and LEGS.)

Pick those YOU want to do. Many can be done any time. Keep them regular to feel THE benefit. NEVER swap exercises about too quickly. Stick to constant schedules.

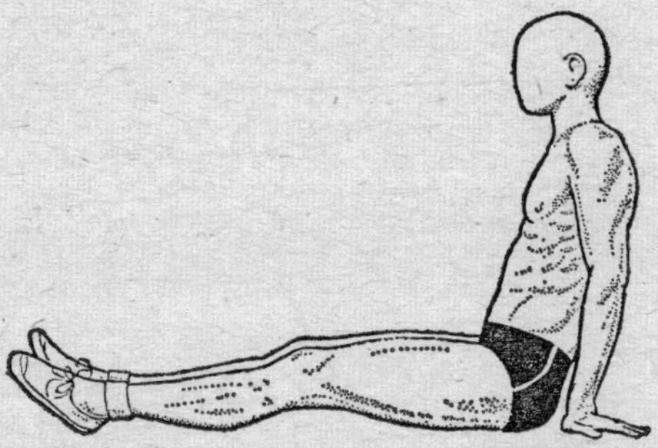

Riser

Sit on floor, legs out and together. Place hands next to hips. Push up lifting glutes/thighs off floor. 10 reps at least a workout.

As you progress: place weight in your lap.

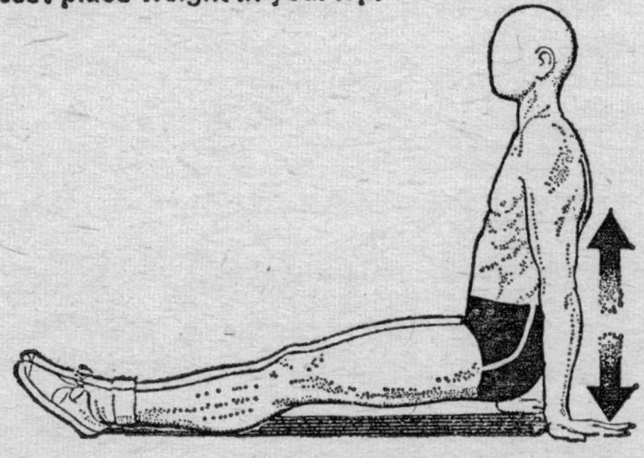

Pushups

Lie prone. Straightarm press straight up from floor (holding back stiff). Then lower to touch nose on mat. No other body part to touch floor.

10 reps = tyro's limit. 30–40 reps = maximum a session for anyone.

Extra resistance = weight (say book) on shoulders.

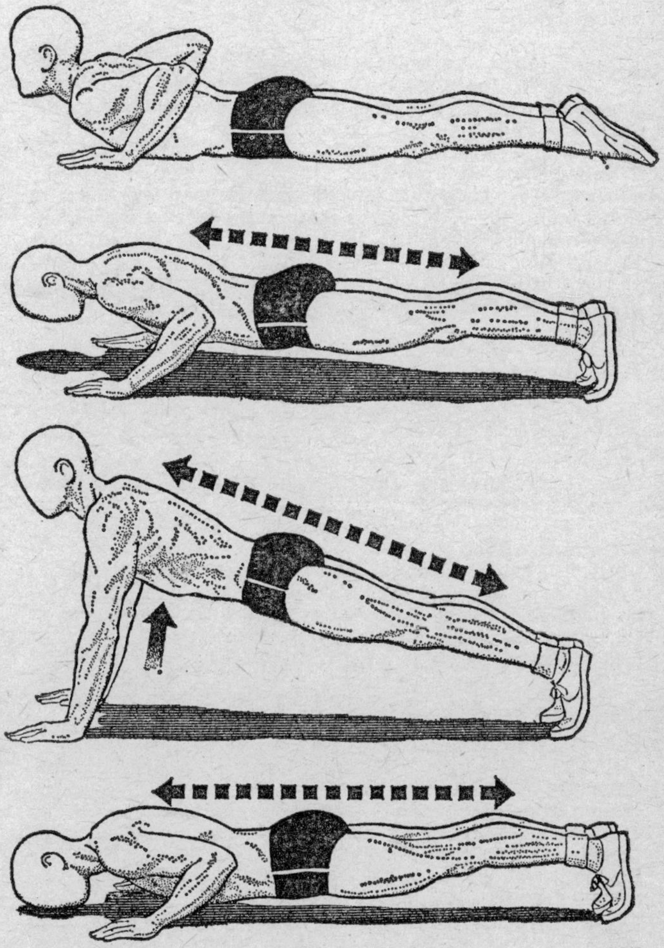

Twister
Hold broom handle in both hands. Step over it. Twist it up and over your back WITHOUT loosening grip or letting handle turn in hands.

Shoulder shover
Stand in doorway palms pressing up under lintel (arms BENT; legs straight). TRY to rocket doortop thro' roof with ARM force for 6 seconds.

THEN . . .

Push hands against jambs (palms on doorposts). Feet astride. Body straight. Toes lined with outside thresh-hold edge. Palms slightly outwards above shoulder level. Raise chest and push/push/push for 6.

Straight arm raise to front
Stand up feet astride on 2 towel ends or on long towel centre. Grasp both ends with fists so pulling taut when arms locked straight/slanting forward at 45 degrees to torso. TRY to raise arms for 6.

Straight arm raise to side
Same thing.

Except locked arms are extended to sides about 45 degrees to torso. Try/try/try to fly. 6 seconds.

Bent forward straight arm raise to side
Bend over from waist still trampling long towel centre. Keep legs/back straight AND arms extended about 45 degrees to sides. Towel ends are grasped. You TRY to PUSHUP torso against towel anchor for 6.

Close grip pullup
Stand feet astride trampling long towel centre. Stand straight. *Elbows* flexed and raised out to sides while fists grip towel ends infront of solar plexus. Breathe in and yank HARD on towel for 6 (forcing shoulder blades together).

Keep elbows OUT.

POURING POWER INTO SHOULDERS

Delts NEED loads of action.

HIT from all angles. YOU need 5 at least of iron-throwing exercises below. At least 2 should feature in regular 6–8 weekly session. Then swapover for *next* 6–8 week period.

General POWer plan = do 3 sets of 8 reps of a PRESSING exercise; AND 3 sets of 12 reps of a LEVERING EXERCISE. Couple new exercises in this way each 6–8 week periods. See below which ARE levering/pressing motions.

Shoulder muscles also worked when doing chest/back/arm

powerpackers. Especially in bench press (see CHEST) and bentover rowing (see BACK).

Press behind neck

As shown.

1. GRASP BARBELL BEHIND NECK (HANDS FAIRLY WIDE APART).
2. PRESS BARBELL TO FULL ARMS' STRETCH ...
3. PUSHING WEIGHT WELL BACK AS IT GOES UPWARDS.

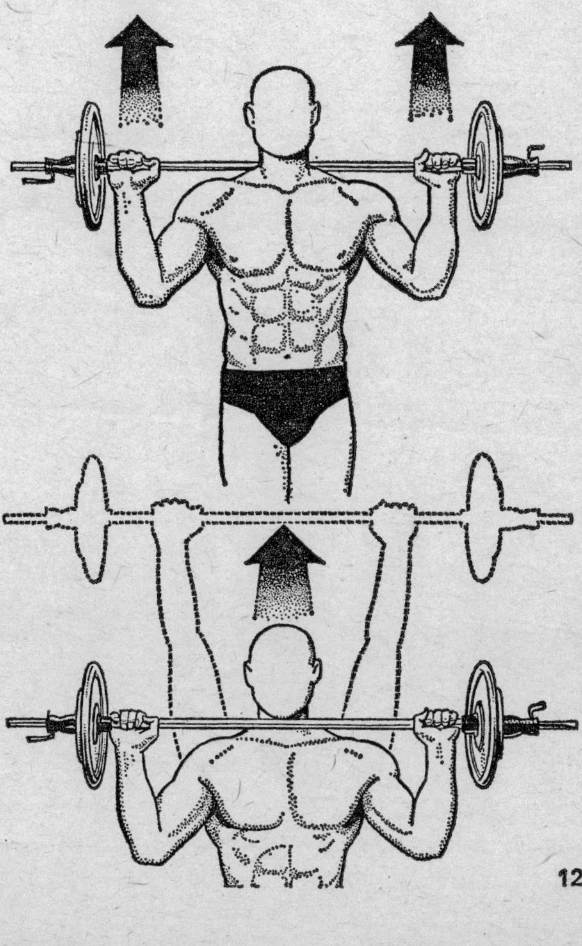

4. LOCK ELBOWS IN STRAIGHT POSITION ON FINAL PUSH.
5. RETURN BAR TO BEHIND HEAD AT START POSITION.

4 sets of 8 reps.

DO this quickly for best results. Stand at first (as sitting press is REAL shoulderburner). Inhale deeply. Don't jerk during movement. NEVER allow bar to rest on shoulders. Remember: too heavy weight will stop you completing reps.
Note: tense ALL body muscles as bar goes up to give extra DRIVE.

Front press
Lift barbell from floor to shoulders (shoulder wide grip) in one movement.* Look upwards for better balance. DRIVE bar in upward press overhead. Relax slightly. Lower bar to shoulders. Tense hard. GO for another rep.

Reps go from shoulder to overhead and back to shoulder again.

**= known as "cleaning" the bar.*

Remember: 6–8 reps in 3 sets for POWer. BUT higher reps for stamina/general fitness.

Seated dumbell press
As shown.

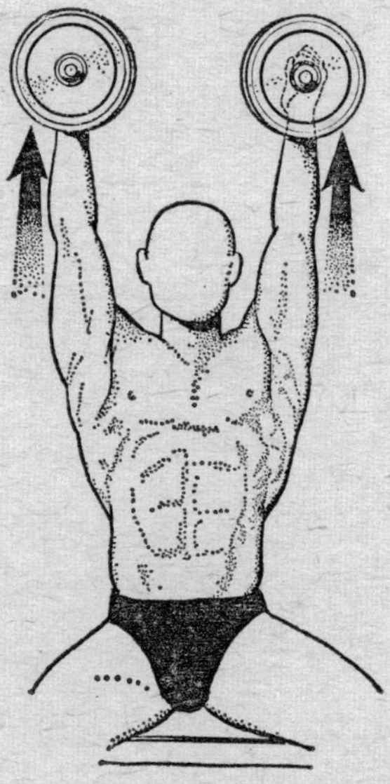

1. SIT EASILY WITH DUMBELL IN EACH FIST HELD TO SHOULDERS, PALMS INWARDS.
2. TAKE DEEP BREATH/BRACE BODY/PRESS DUMBELLS TO . . .
3. FULL ARMS STRETCH OVERHEAD.
4. PAUSE BRIEFLY.
5. LOWER BELLS TO SHOULDERS READY FOR NEXT REP.

3 sets of 8 reps.

Note: do NOT lean back from waist. Be sure to press weights *back* as they travel UP.

Barbell pullovers

Lie on floor holding barbell behind head. Pull them over chest, dip them down to chest, press back up, THEN lower to thighs. Lift barbells from thighs back to behind head (for best results).

And repeat.

One arm press

As shown.

1. CLEAN* BELLS TO SHOULDERS.
2. ALTERNATELY PRESS THEM OVERHEAD IN POWERFUL PUSHES.

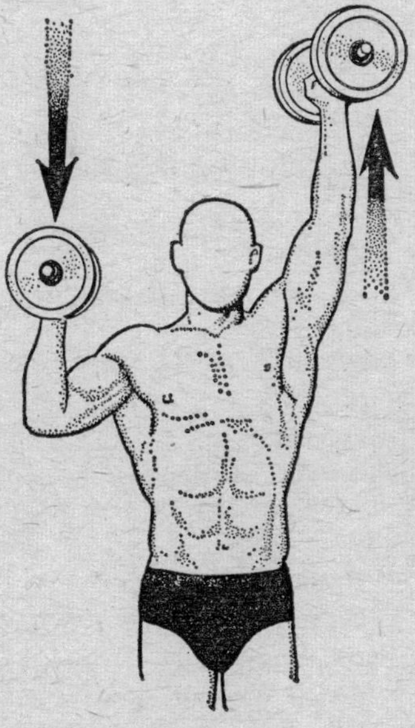

3. EXHALING AS EACH BELL IS ON UP STROKE, INHALING AS LOWERED.

*= *see p.* 146.

Note: take care to keep control of this testing exercise. IF you can press 100 lbs. barbell it does not mean you can press 50 lbs. with *each* hand.

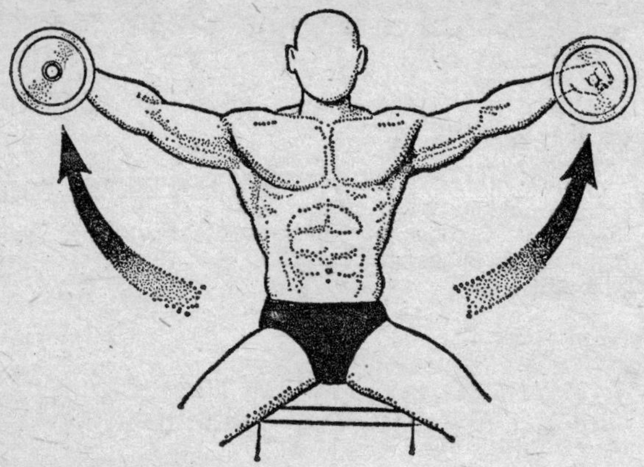

Seated lateral raise

As shown.

Sit down. Use light dumbells.

1. GRASP DUMBELLS (10-POUNDERS).
2. SIT BACK-STRAIGHT ACROSS BENCH ALLOWING ARMS TO HANG.
3. KEEPING TRUNK STRAIGHT, STEADILY RAISE ARMS OUT TO SIDE AND UP . . .
4. UNTIL IN LINE WITH SHOULDERS (OR OVERHEAD).
5. PAUSE BRIEFLY AND . . .
6. LOWER SLOWLY SO ARMS COME TO SIDES (UNDER CONTROL).

3 sets of 8 reps.

Note: concentrate/concentrate/concentrate. Breathe in as weights raised, out as lowered. Keep body tense all time weights come down (by tightening grip).

Bentover lateral raise

As shown.

1. STAND FEET APART, DUMBELL IN EACH FIST.
2. BEND OVER UNTIL TORSO = PARALLEL TO FLOOR (REST HEAD ON TABLE).

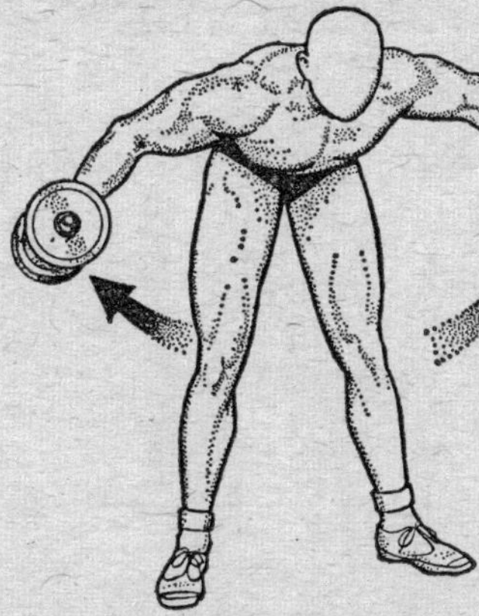

3. DROP ARMS STRAIGHT SO DUMBELLS NEAR FLOOR AND SLIGHTLY BEND KNEES.
4. WITHOUT SWINGING RAISE DUMBELLS SIDEWAYS AND BACKWARDS UNTIL HIGHER THAN BACK.
5. HOLD FOR A SECOND. THEN LOWER.

Take it slowly.

Standing sideways lateral raise
Stand feet apart, arms hanging, clutching bells (palms in). Raise them until shoulder level. Hold for moment. Lower to thighs.

Forward raise
Take same START position as above (dumbells at hang). But raise dumbells FORWARD to shoulder level. Hold for a second then return to thighs.

Can be done with barbell in same way.

Shoulder shrug
Hold barbell in hang position across pelvis (arms at shoulder width; palms towards you). Shrug/lower shoulders. AS you shrug shoulders ALSO pull them backwards.

Upright rowing
As shown.

1. GRIP BARBELL WITH 4 in. HAND SPACING/HANDS HANGING DOWN BODY/KNUCKLES TO FRONT.
2. ENERGETICALLY YANK BAR UP TO NECK LEVEL AND ...

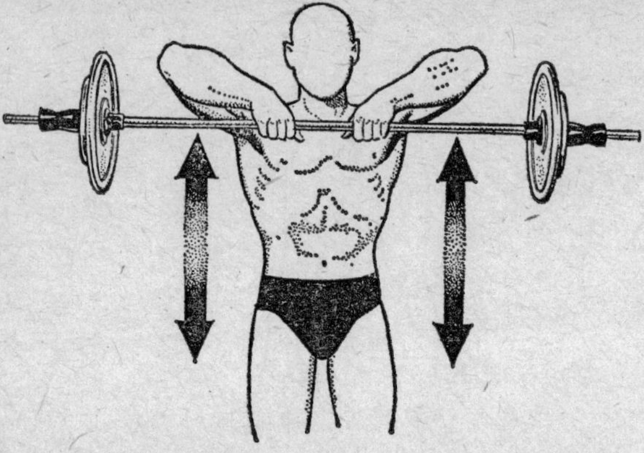

3. RAISE ELBOWS HIGH.*
4. KEEP BAR CLOSE TO BODY WHILE RAISING.
4. AND FIGHT NOT TO LEANBACK FROM WAIST.
6. LOWER/REPEAT.

3 sets of 10.
*= *wrists do NOT turn over.*

Alternate forward raise
(Similar to holding weight to front strength test: see earlier in SHOULDERS.)

1. STAND PRESSING HEELS/GLUTES/SHOULDERS TO WALL.
2. LIGHT DUMBELL IS GRIPPED IN EACH FIST (KNUCKLES FORWARD).
3. ALTERNATELY RAISE THEM TO OVERHEAD.
4. PAUSE BRIEFLY THEN ...
5. LOWER SLOWLY/DELIBERATELY/LOOKING UP.

3 sets of 8.
DO make it rythmic. Breathe naturally through mouth.

AND TWO POWERGIVERS WITH READYFOUND GEAR

Chairswinger

As shown opposite.

Hold kitchen chair lightly at lower part of backrest. Use tips of curled fingers. Swing chair up WITH arms straight for 10-count.
10 reps working up to 25 (AND holdout chair longer too).

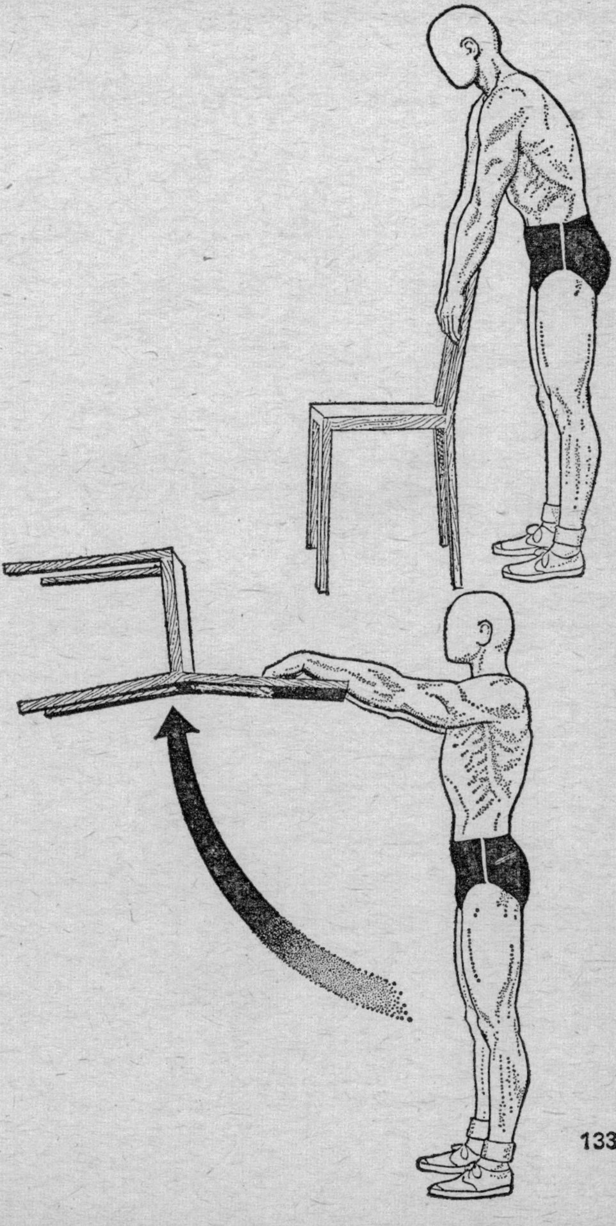

Inner tube stretcher

As shown.

Stretch tube behind back. Swing arms forward. And pump arms forwards/backwards combating S-T-R-E-T-C-H.

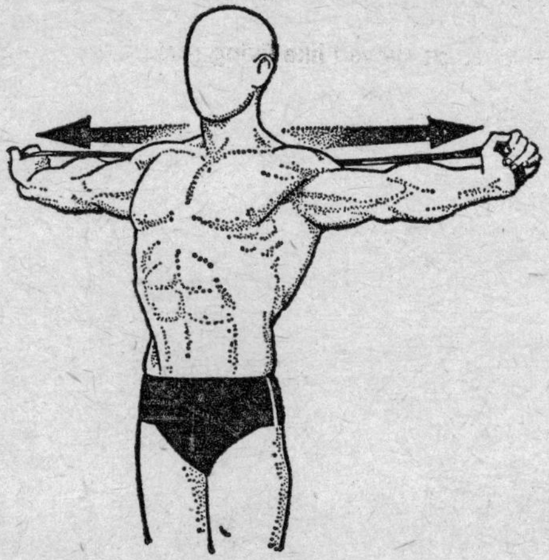

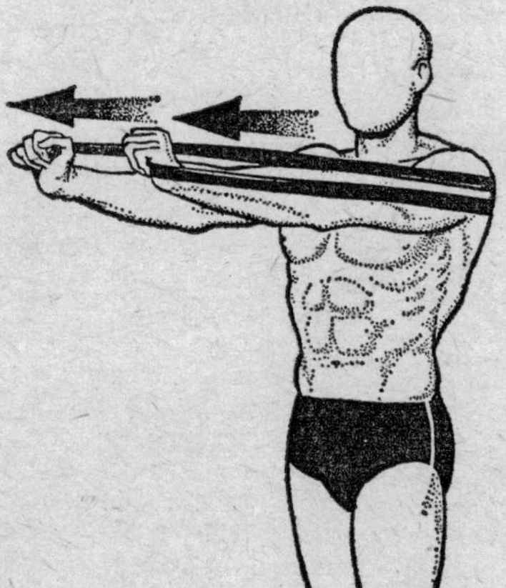

BACK

YOUR BACK is cornerstone of STRENGTH. A weak back = A weak YOU. Unable to take advantage of existing leg power YOU have weakest link in potential Herculean chain. All men need a shockproof back for lifting/shoving/manhandling. Yet true and rugged exercise will give YOU a 100-megaton hindside stuffed with strength from lower waist to shoulder top. With lats that funnel torso from armpits to waistband, traps to add to shoulder line and muscle columns sandwiching lower spine . . . YOUR back can be hewed like living rock from to-day.

PACK BACK POWER NOW

By lifting/pushing MR TOUGH's way.

Lift a BIG man
With Fireman's lift (as shown).

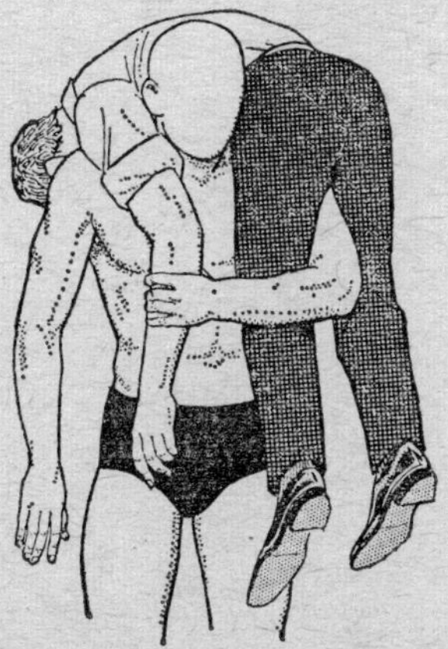

Practice first: threading right/left arm between his legs, gripping his wrist on same side of body with YOUR other hand, and LIFTING with leg/back power.

Man is easily carried. Like potatoes sack.

Carry 50 lbs. uphill
And much more if already strong.

By making packframe (as shown). Use bit of old board + webbing straps + cord. Lash load to board.* Carry this HIGH on shoulders using webbing for shoulderstraps. Keep load well clear of hips/kidneys/small of back. AND it will FLOAT along (superior to rucksack carrying).

*= *make small ledge at bottom of board to prevent load*

slipping. Instead of a board you CAN make a frame if preferred.
Tie broad cloth band to top of packframe with cord. Wear band round brow to ease load with neck muscle help.

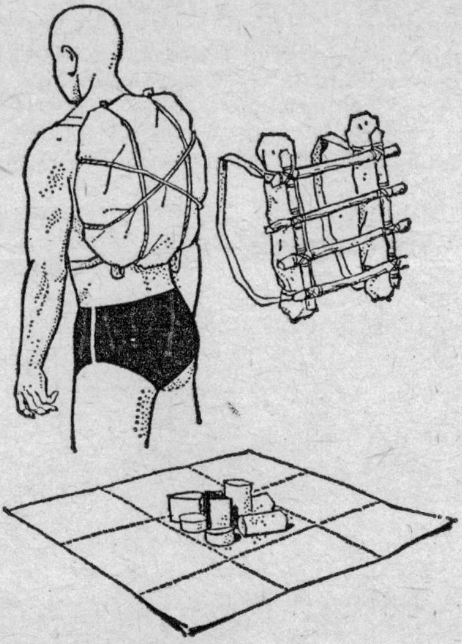

Lift a boulder off the deck
Bend knees, crouching. Tug load on to your toes. This lets fingers slide underneath. Lift rock on to knees, sliding forearms underneath. Stand up (back straight), legs giving POWer. Hoist rock to chest. Curl fingers at far side.
Note: breathe freely; don't try BIG boulders at first (work up from small ones). NEVER jerk/strain/sprain. THINK. Then lift smoothly.

Bend your KNEES rather than SPINE. Back should be /-shape or !-shape. NEVER ?-shape.

Giant stones CAN be moved by lifting one edge, then rolling while YOU balance rock upright for a few feet under its own momentum.
Warning: watch your toes.

Manoeuvre a log
Use boulder lift + cunning.

1. GRIP LOGEND/BEND KNEES/KEEP BACK STRAIGHT.
2. LIFT AND . . .
3. WALK CRABWISE SIDESTEPPING.

4. THEN LOWER THAT END SLOWLY.
5. GO TO OTHER LOGEND AND LIFT THAT UNTIL ...
6. YOU CAN CARRY IT PAST THE FAR END.
7. REPEAT ENDS UNTIL LOG IS IN POSITION.

Remember: bend knees and keep back straight on LOWERING too.

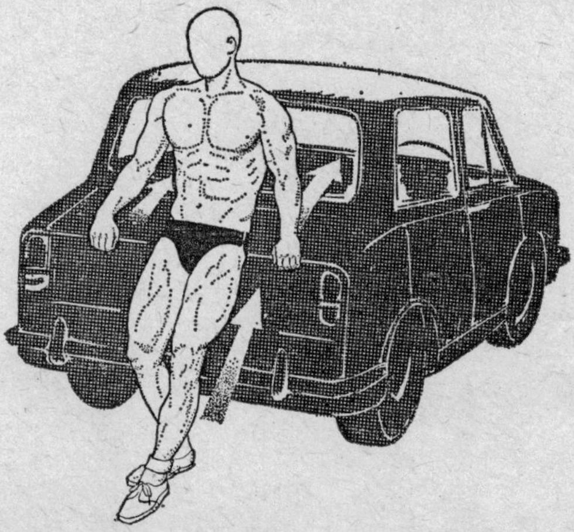

Shove sticking car/van/truck

As shown.

1. JOCKEY BACK TO VEHICLE WITH ...
2. LEGS AT 45 DEGREES TO THE GROUND.
3. BEND KNEES/DIG HEELS IN/AND ...
4. DRIVE WITH LEGPOWER AS YOU STRAIGHTEN THEM.

Repeat bending/straightening legs.

DAILY BACK TONERS

For a fine straight back with impressive nonmilitary BUT definitely man-of-power bearing.

Almost *all* exercises with/without weights will muscleup BACK to some degree. Help these further with specialist grafters.

Bar chinning

(See also ARMS.)

As shown overleaf.

Reach up for bar/lintel/branch. Grasp with handpalms towards you. Hands little more than shoulder width apart. Pullup to touch bar with chin. Slowly lower to full arms' stretch.

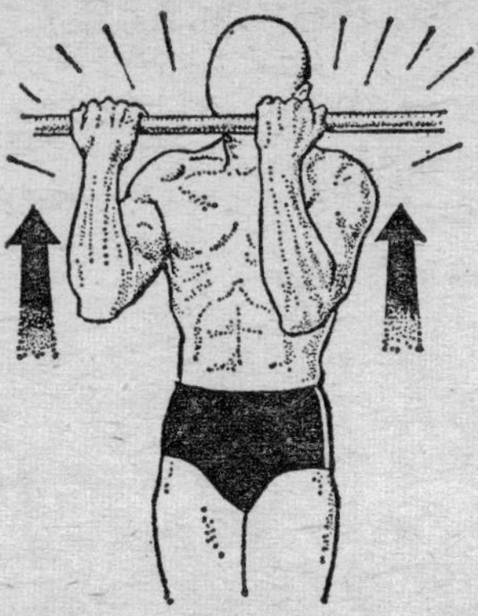

Lower slowly. NEVER *drop.* Heavily built find this rough exercise; lightweights find it easier.

Start with 6 reps. Work up to 12–15.

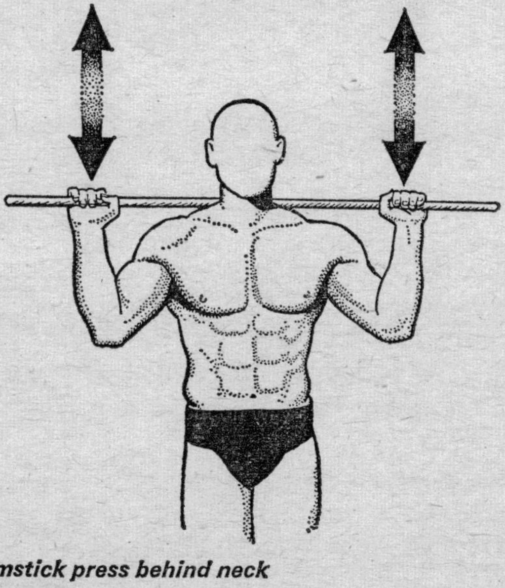

Broomstick press behind neck

As shown.

Take broomstick above head. Now bring bar down behind

neck. Breathe in through mouth. Now push bar back to start position. Smoothly.

3 sets of 10 (if over 45 try 4 sets of 6).

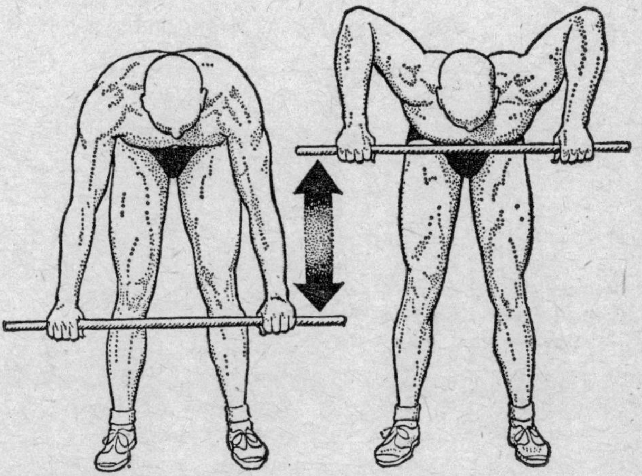

Bentforward rowing with broomstick

As shown.

1. STAND STRAIGHT HOLDING HANDLE JUST OUTSIDE SHOULDER WIDTH.
2. BEND FORWARD TORSO PARALLEL TO FLOOR, ARMS DROPPING.
3. BRING HANDLE TO CHEST TAKING DEEP BREATH.
4. PUSH HANDLE BACK DOWN TO FULL ARMS DROP, EXHALING.
5. SWING IT/TRUNK STILL/ONLY ARMS WORKING.
6. AND TRUNK KEPT BENT.

3 sets of 20 (if over 45 try 3 sets of 10).

Stifflegged deadlift with broomstick

As shown overleaf.

1. HOLD BROOMHANDLE IN BENT FORWARD POSITION (TORSO PARALLEL TO FLOOR).
2. BREATHE IN AS YOU RISE UP MAKING SHOULDERS GO RIGHT BACK.
3. NOW BEND FORWARD BREATHING OUT.

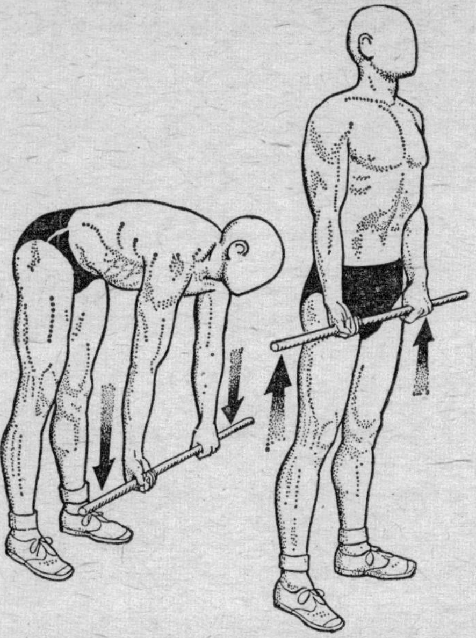

4. KEEPING LEGS STRAIGHT THROUGHOUT MOVEMENT.

Note: one fist should face forward, other backwards (see later why).

BACKPACK INSTANT MICROPOWER

Anywhere/anytime/anyone. Do 6 seconds a shot.

Shrug spoiler

Sit well forward on chair. Feet together and flat on floor. Don't lean forward. DO grip with fingers and handpalms under each thigh midway along. Sit straight. TRY to shrug shoulders. Only don't let thighgrab allow it.

Lower prone back spoiler

Lie face down with heels under bed. Fold arms infront of you. Breathe in. TRY to LIFT object through roof with heels. Keeping legs straight and lifting from hips. 6 seconds.

Spinal stretcher

Sit on floor knees up. Round back. Stretch forward. Grasp

ankles. IF arms not full stretched push away feet until they are. Take deep breath and PULL back. 6 seconds fight.

Towel shrug
Stand trampling long towel so arms straight down by sides. Grip each towelend firmly. Inhale deeply. TRY to shrug shoulders against towel opposition. 6 seconds.

Trunk raise
Trample long towel under feet (about 18 in. apart). Grip ends after bending forward so torso = parallel to floor. Hang arms straight down towards feet. Hold towel taut (above kneecap level). TRY to raise upper body with big tussle. Lock legs throughout this movement. NEVER pull with arms; let trunk muscles do the work.

Trunk raise with more towels
Same exercise as trunk raise BUT drape another towel round neck (as well as other towel YOU are trampling underfoot). Ball fists to clench 2 towelends each when bent forward (as shown). TRY to forceup trunk for 6 seconds.

Tugback
Sit on floor with legs straight out (flat on floor). Put towel round feetsoles and grip ends with fists (about thigh position). Round YOUR back. Pull tight with fully stretched arms. Inhale first. Toss back head. Resist with legpower to stop leanback.

Straight arm press down to side
Sit/stand with one arm at shoulder level pressing on flat furniture surface (straightout). Press down HARD for 6 seconds. Swap hands.
Note: arm MUST be parallel to floor. Arm locked at elbow. And forced down level with shoulders.

Bent forward press down to side
Bend forward until torso = parallel to floor, Keep legs/back straight. Raise arms straight out to side AND force handpalms down on tabletop. IF hard to arrange 2-handed press DO one hand at a time.

PACK BACK WITH IRON POWER

Work HARD.

Generally in 6–8 week programme: DO one exercise for upper back, one for lower. 3 sets each. IF specialising in back development do 2 upper and 2 lower back movements. Memo: low reps for POWer/bulk; high reps for stamina.

Again: ALL standing up exercises packpower into BACK. BUT you need that bit extra for body hindside as mostly BIG muscles here.

LOWER BACK POWERING

Very important: don't neglect for REAL power.

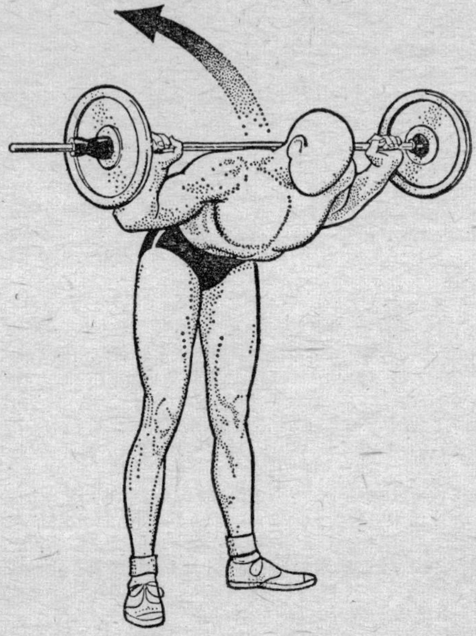

Good Morning exercise

As shown.

1. STAND FEET ASTRIDE, BARBELL ACROSS TOWEL-PADDED NECKNAPE.
2. BEND FORWARD FROM HIPS UNTIL TORSO PARALLEL TO FLOOR.
3. KEEPING LEGS STIFF.
4. COME ERECT AND REPEAT.

Breathe out on way down; in as you come up.

Deadlift

As shown.

A classic (*stifflegged*). One of THE big 3 (along with squats/bench press). Also great for upper back powering.
Note: use good poundage from very start; try $1\frac{1}{2}$ times own body weight and see how things go.

1. STAND FEET APART, BARBELL ON FLOOR INFRONT OF TOES.

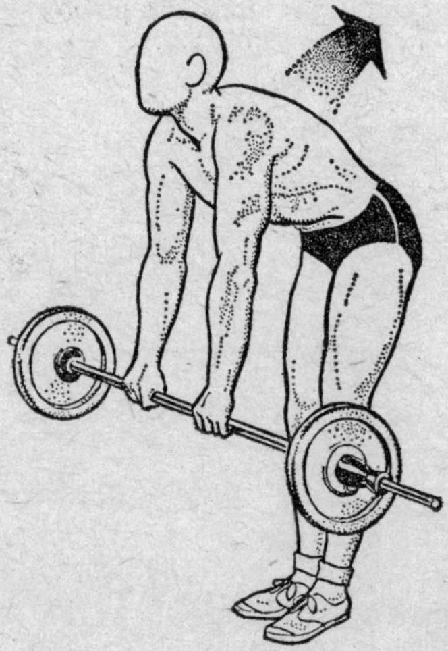

2. BEND AT WAIST AND GRASP BAR WITH SHOULDER-WIDE GRIP.
3. KEEPING LEGS STIFF PULL BAR UP BY STRAIGHTENING BACK.
4. DO NOT BEND ARMS TO GET BAR HIGHER.
5. ARMS REMAIN STRAIGHT AT ALL TIMES.

As you come erect inhale lifting chest high. AND tug shoulders well back. Exhale as YOU lower bar to floor.

Note: *can* be done with legs slightly bent (straighten them as weight lifted). THIS is *standard* deadlift. DO it this way if BACK is weak now (so you employ legpower to help out).

3 sets of 10.

Hyper extension exercise

Excellent for lower back.

As shown overleaf

Lie face down across training bench with mate gripping feet by ankles (SO only thightops/lower abs balances on training bench. Clasp hands behind neck. Arch back. Rise back up as shown.

Lower torso to floor. Then (by towing with erector spinae muscles) pull torso back up to start position. Breathe in as back is arched, out as body is lowered.

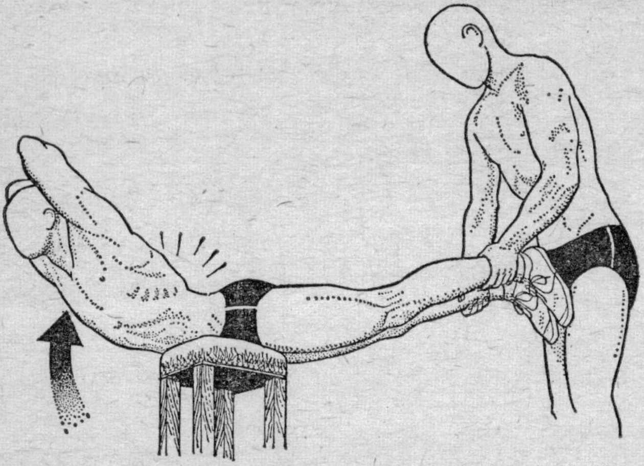

IRON POWER FOR YOUR UPPER BACK

Pack those lats/traps with STRENGTH.

Chinning bars

As in prepower exercises. BUT to a definite routine HERE as brawnyback-maker.

Grasp overhead bar so body hangs full stretch (kick-a-chair-away/jumpup/climbup or any other manoeuvre so YOU can *hang* straightout from high bar).

Have hands little more than shoulder width apart. PULLUP *hard* to chin bar. Or as near as you can. NOW lower to full arms stretch and PULLUP again without stopping. Breathe out as you go UP, IN as you descend.

Do it both with knuckles forwards AND backwards. Front facing knuckles + narrow handgrip = good for ARMS too.

TRY chinning smoothly as possible. Without tugging/straining/wrestling. Do as many as can for 3 sets with 60 seconds rest inbetween.

Chinning behind neck

1. HANG FROM BAR WITH HANDPALMS AWAY FROM YOU.
2. AND ARMS STRAIGHT.
3. PULL UP AS FOR BAR CHINNING BUT ...
4. NOD HEAD AND TRY TO TOUCH BAR WITH NECK-NAPE.
5. LOWER AND REPEAT.

HARD exercise (but piles on strength *fast*). Use very wide handgrip. Do most possible for 3 sets with 60 seconds break inbetween.

10 reps = YOU can start thinking about adding extra weight to waist (hang old iron from belt).

Barbell bentover rowing

As with broomstick (see earlier).

1. STAND WITH FEET ASTRIDE AND GRASP BARBELL WITH FAIRLY WIDE GRIP.
2. LEAN FORWARD FROM WAIST ALLOWING ARMS TO HANG STRAIGHT DOWN.
3. KEEP BACK FLAT.
4. GIVE HUGE HEAVE AND YANK BAR UP TO TOUCH CHEST THEN ...
5. LOWER IT TO STRAIGHT ARMS DOWN AGAIN.

Sway body a little to keep weight in motion (especially when weight is heavy). BUT never overdo bodysway or YOU rob BACK of POWerchance. Breathe in as bar is raised; out as lowered.

3 sets of 12.

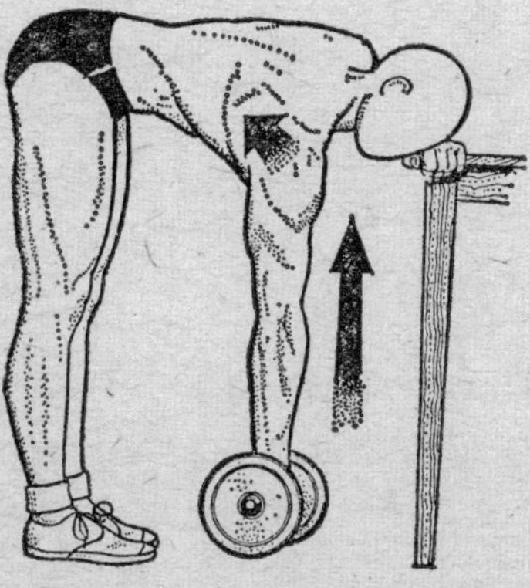

Single arm rowing with dumbells

As shown.

1. KEEP BACK/LEGS STRAIGHT AS YOU REST HEAD ON FOREARM (HAND PRESSING ON TABLE/STOOL/CHAIRBACK).
2. GRASP DUMBELL IN OTHER HAND ABOUT 1 in. FROM FLOOR.

3. RAISE THAT ELBOW VERY HIGH TO PULL DUMBELL UP TO SHOULDER AND ...
4. SHRUG SHOULDER GIRDLE WELL BACK.
5. LOWER WEIGHT BACK TO START CONTROLLING IT ALL THE WAY.

Lock head solid across arm. Use heavy dumbell to = REAL work.

3 sets of 12 reps an arm (alternate sets per arm).

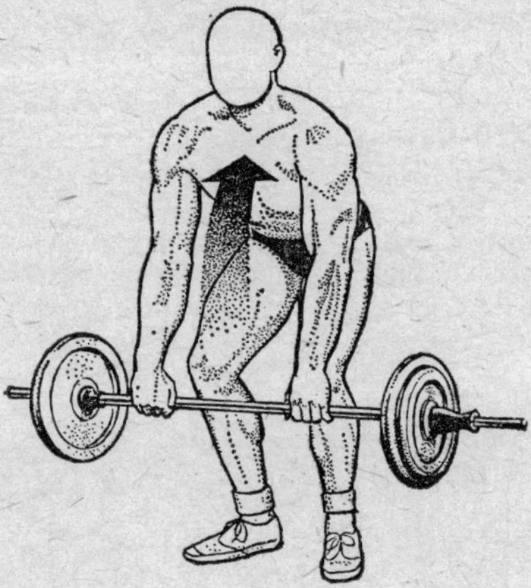

The clean

THIS = Part 1 of an Olympic lift BUT great for MR TOUGH too.

As shown.

1. STAND KNEES BENT/BACK FLAT/HEAD UP AND ...
2. PALMS IN AS YOU GRIP BARBELL ACROSS SHINS WITH ...
3. JUST - OVER - SHOULDER - WIDTH - GRASP, ARMS STRAIGHT.
4. NOW ...
5. STRAIGHTEN LEGS WITH POWER AND WHIP UP BAR TO CHEST.
6. AS BAR PASSES CHEST HEIGHT, BEND LEGS TO ...
7. LOWER YOUR BODY AGAIN AND LET YOU GET UNDER BAR.

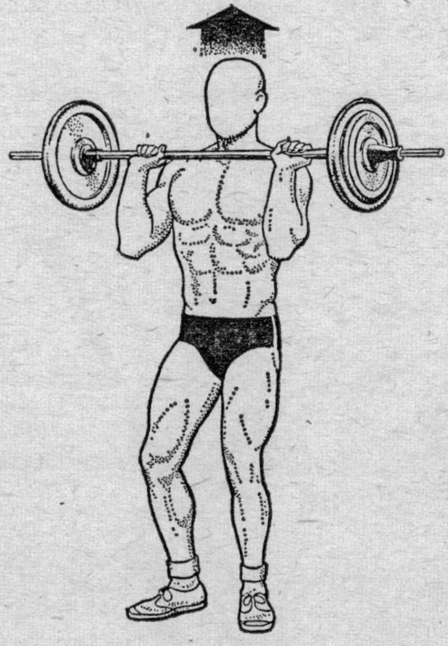

8. TURNOVER HANDS AT WRISTS AS BAR COMES TO REST AT SHOULDERS.
9. COME ERECT WITH BAR BY STRAIGHTENING LEGS TO COMPLETE MOVEMENT.

Clean is excellent warmingup exercise. Use only 50 per cent poundage from what YOU can manage to warmup muscle in advance.

READYFOUND POWERPACKERS FOR BACK

Slot these in with Iron throwing.

As shown overleaf.

INNER TUBE YANKER: cross inner tubes from each foot to opposite fists. Keep pulling.

INNER TUBE EXPANDER: sit and loop inner tubes over feet AND handbacks. Now pull hard. Stretch tubes as far as possible.

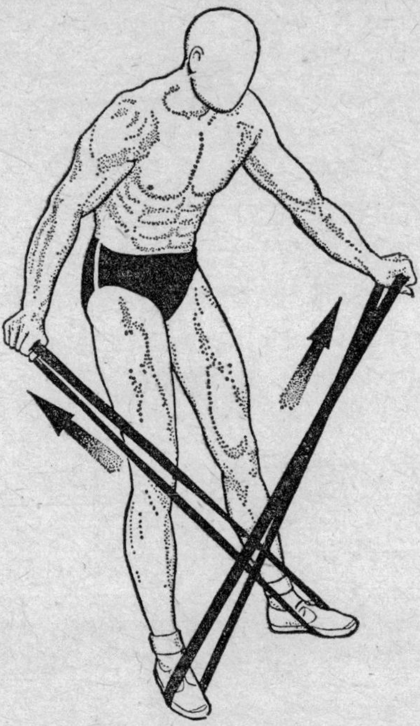

Inner tube yanker

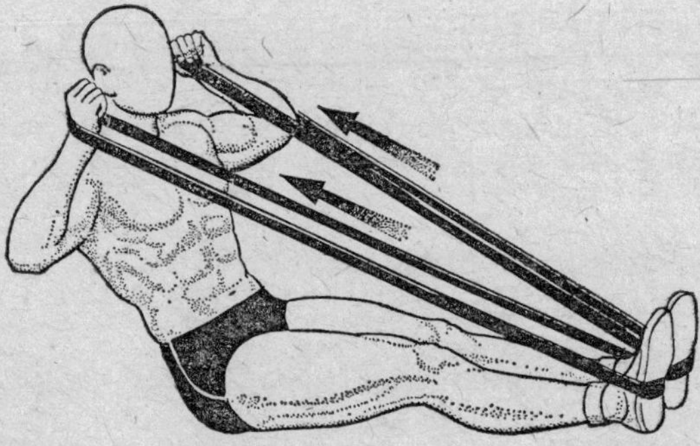

Inner tube expander

SANDBAG FLYER: raise sandbag in each hand straight out from sides. Hold at arms' length as long as possible. Lower slowly. At least 5 reps daily.

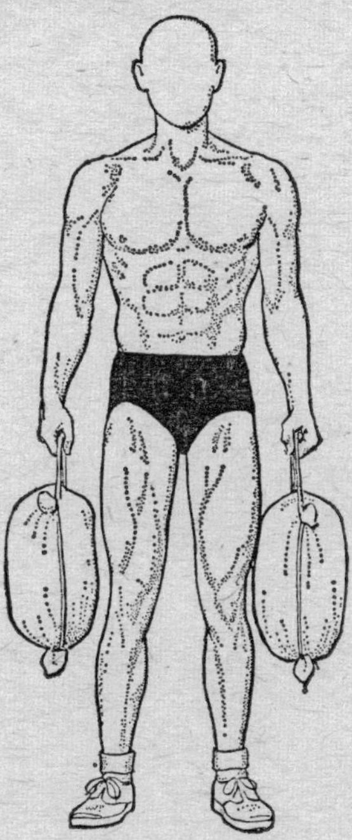

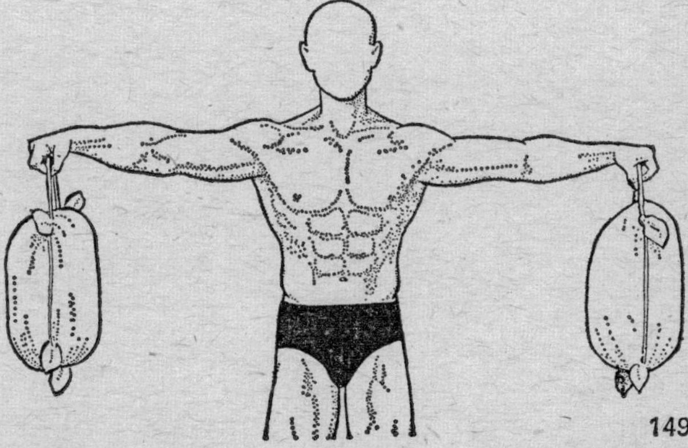

FINGERS/HANDS/WRISTS

FINGERS/HANDS/WRISTS: 6

YOUR HANDS are the most marvellous machines *never* invented. Nothing ever devised by man can take their place. YOU use hands 1,000's of times more than any other body part daily. And in 100's of ways.

Powerful grip = powerful man. Whether crushing bones with a handshake or wresting off bottle caps no one else can shift, YOUR fists can gain instant respect. Punch home the strength that 20 forearm muscles hand to YOU.

Make puttysoft hands ironhard/velvet-toned/glovesupple (never hamfisted). ALREADY you are stronger-fingered than you think (and can prove it immediately). MR TOUGH will double that grip in weeks.

WHAT FINGERS AND HANDS WILL DO NOW

Use knack to handout finger power. Try handstrength feats as tests (making feats harder + succeeding = knowing hands gaining strength).

Fire fingers like bullets

Place dry beer mat over ½-pint glass.

As shown overleaf.

1. POISE FIST ABOVE, 2nd FINGER DOWN STIFF.
2. CHECK FINGER AT 90 DEGREES TO MAT.
3. SHOOT FINGER STRAIGHT FOR MAT AND ...
4. PIERCE THROUGH IT.

All men can drill ONE mat (and two with practice). Three

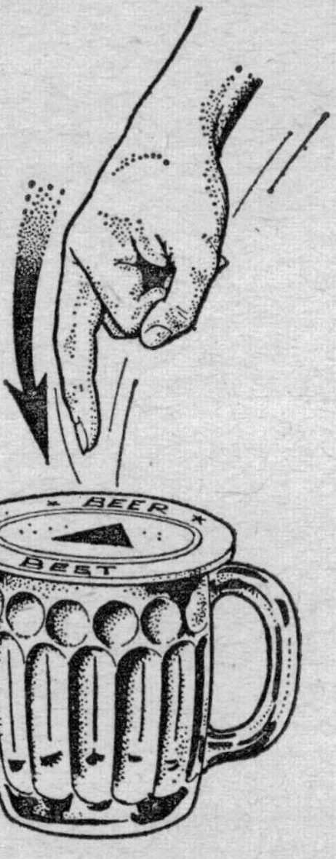

mats = golden bullseye of finger power (and possible to YOU).

BUT *scrap inhibition which fires blanks.* Think of mat 3 feet lower than it is so finger meets it *full blast.*

Make sledgehammer fist

Sharpen 6 in. nail end beesting sharp. Span thinnest plank of soft wood (like pine) *level* between 2 chairs/tables/stools. Ball nail head in thick duster as shock absorber to fit hand palm.
As shown opposite.

1. CAREFULLY LOCK PROTRUDING NAIL BETWEEN 1st/2nd or 2nd/3rd FINGERS.
2. SEAT HEAD FIRMLY IN HAND CENTRE.
3. RAISE HAND.
4. CONCENTRATE ON THAT BOARD/HATE IT/KILL IT WITH . . .
5. MIGHTY BLOW OF FIST + NAIL.

Nail smashes thro' board like cheese. Soon—a wouldbe MR TOUGH can bash past 1 in. planks.

Note: nail MUST be arrow straight in 90 degree fireline. Also:

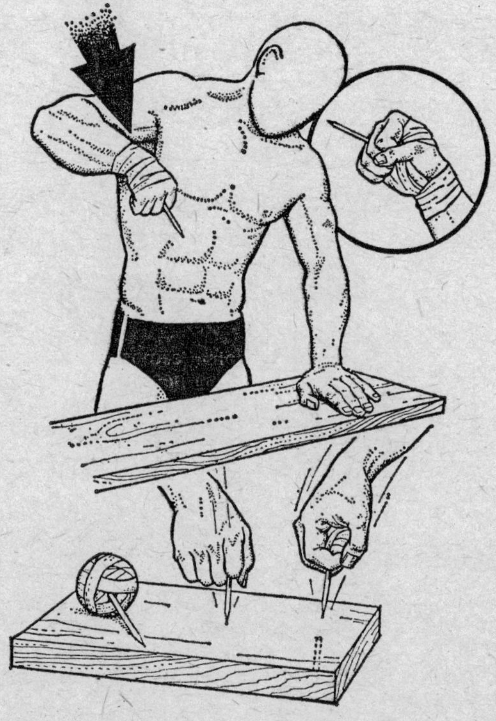

balled duster can be bound into palm with bandage (as shown).

Beat strongest man you know in test of strength
As shown overleaf.

Stand facing, hands up.

1. INTERLOCK FINGERS AT CHEST LEVEL.
2. READY/STEADY/GO!
3. GRAPPLE FOR SUBMISSION.
4. PRESS AT BASE OF OPPONENTS LITTLE FINGERS WITH YOUR 3rd FINGERS.
5. AND TURN ALL YOUR FINGERTIPS OUTWARDS SAME WAY.

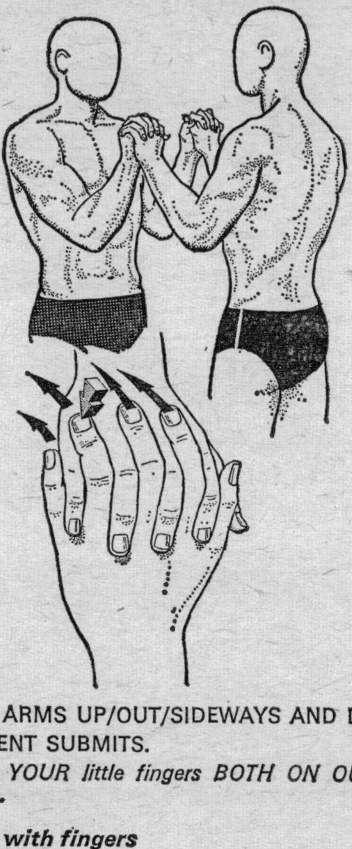

6. SWING ARMS UP/OUT/SIDEWAYS AND DOWN.
7. OPPONENT SUBMITS.

**= ensure YOUR little fingers BOTH ON OUTSIDE of finger mesh.*

Scissor string with fingers

Do as shown opposite.

Diag. 154

Any string does from gardening to twine. Try on weakest first. Check 2–3 feet of slack to give extra savage jerk. Remember: have string near root of fingers for maximum power.

Combat fiercest handshake

Give strong one yourself by sliding hand *right forward* (extended forefinger = extra foil). Best way to give power handshake = try pincer grip exercises (see later).

Gaze straight at handcrusher at oneup point:

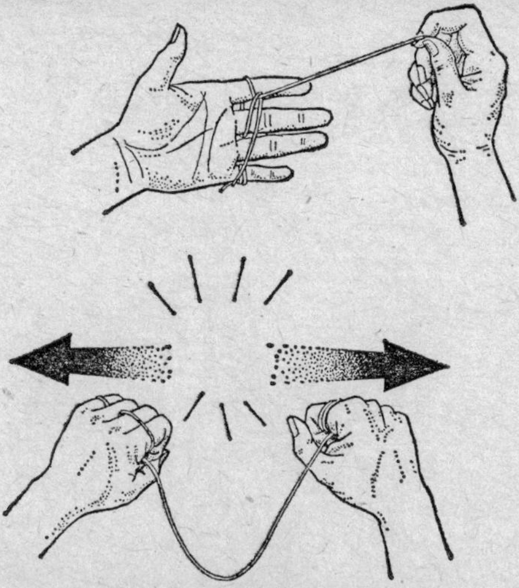

Open up beer bottles barehanded
Hold pair in grip as shown. And lever with flip action.

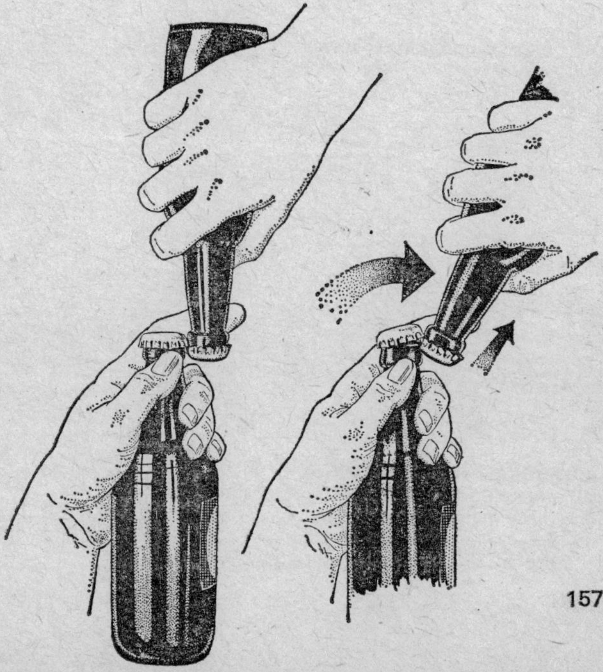

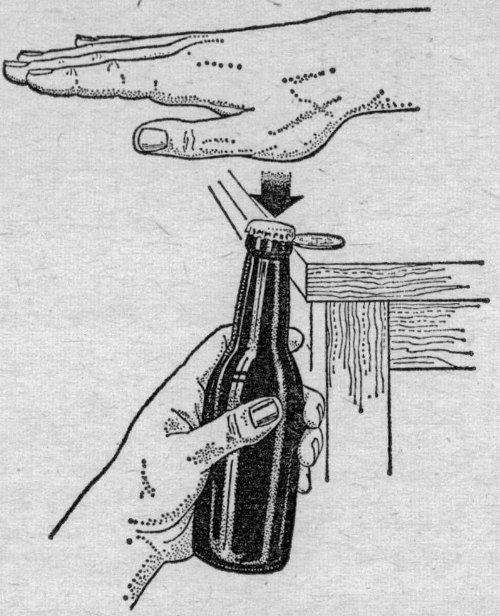

1 bottle can·be done this way.

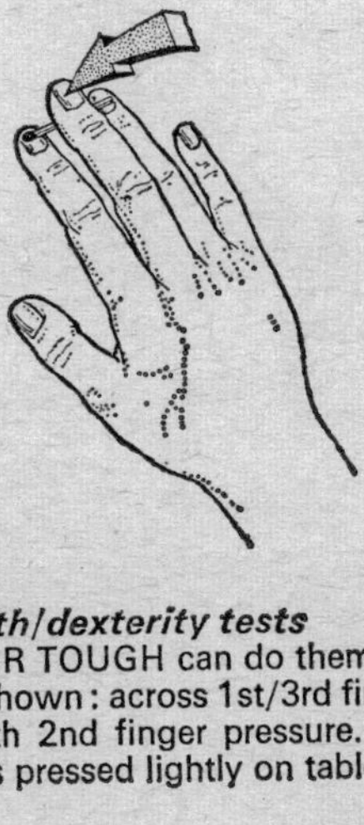

Matchstick strength/dexterity tests

Both are hard. But MR TOUGH can do them.

(a) Place match as shown: across 1st/3rd finger and under 2nd. Try to cut it with 2nd finger pressure. Cheat at first with bottom fingertips pressed lightly on table.

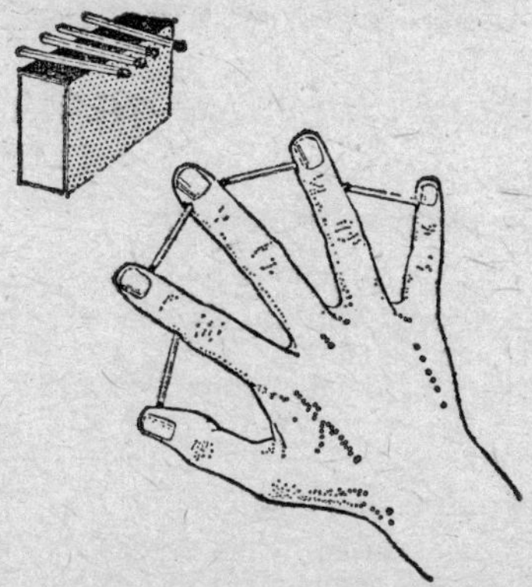

(b) Place 8 matches as shown across matchbox side. Then try for 1 match to span gap between *each* finger and thumb. Supple strength wins.

Rip pack of cards in half

Harder than telephone directory bisection BUT soon OK with practice on old bits of cardboard.

1. BEND DECK VIGOROUSLY TO MACHINEGUN RIP-LINE FIBRES.
2. STICK DECK UPRIGHT IN ONE PALM AND GRAB FIRMLY.

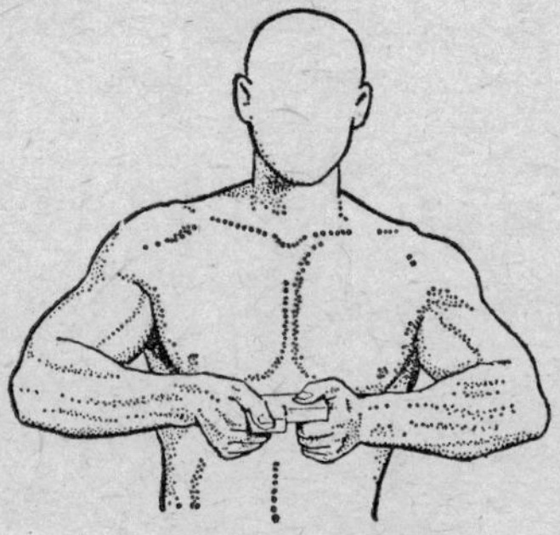

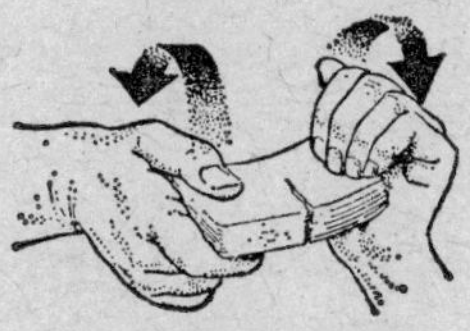

3. COVER OTHER END WITH OTHER HAND AND GRIP TOO.
4. TWIST UNDERHAND UP AND OVERHAND DOWN.
5. KEEP IT UP UNTIL . . .
6. PACK SEVERED WITH GRUNT.

Vital point = fan cards slightly (a la telephone book) as hands wrestle cards back/forth with top and under hand. Start deck rip one card at a time therefore.

Best training workout = squeezing rubber ball.

Straphang from an empty fist

Pick boulder by roadside with thin vertical crack running up *smooth* rock. Challenge companion to climb it. Then prove it possible: by inserting hand, slotting thumb across palm (as shown) and using swelling hand as hand grip to lift you up climberstyle. Practice first.

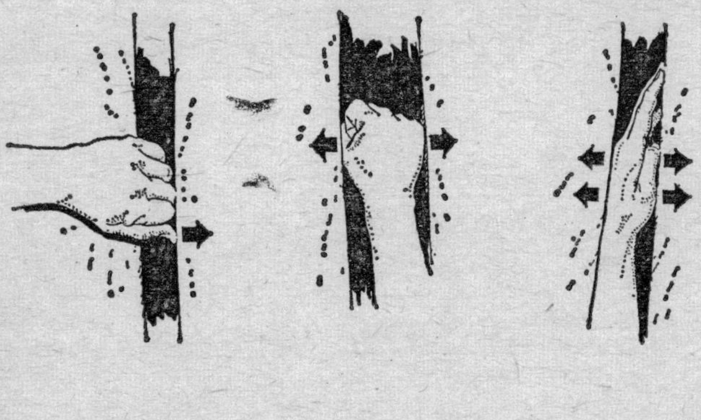

MAKE THE BEST OF YOUR HANDS IMMEDIATELY

Cut fingernails straight across. Brush nail dirt out (NOT scrape it). Press nails with fingertips to = good cuticles. Scrap wearing gloves unless very cold.

Tetanus injection saves YOU from rusty tin can cut risks (hands vulnerable).

Keep wrists straight pushing/lifting/shoving. Fist = very strong when curled up; weak turned down (as in thumbs down position). Straight wrists = full power.

All men can karate chop planks/bricks/etc. AFTER karate training in (1) making superb fist, (2) losing inhibition. Practice fist manufacture NOW (as shown). Go for TIGHT fist. Thumb outside and pressed down tightly. Takes years of practice.

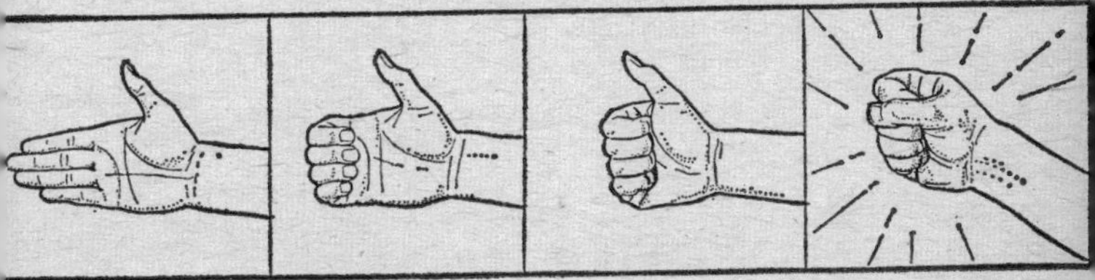

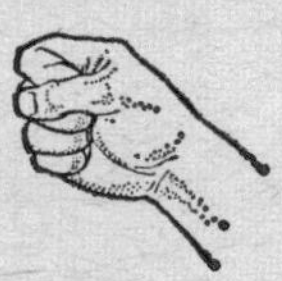

Yes.

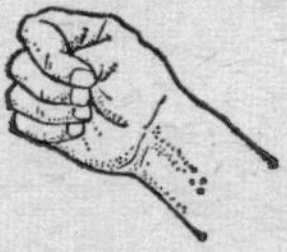

No.

If you *have* to use fist TRY to start blow at hips with palm side of the fist upwards. Twist fist as it comes up. Hit palm-side

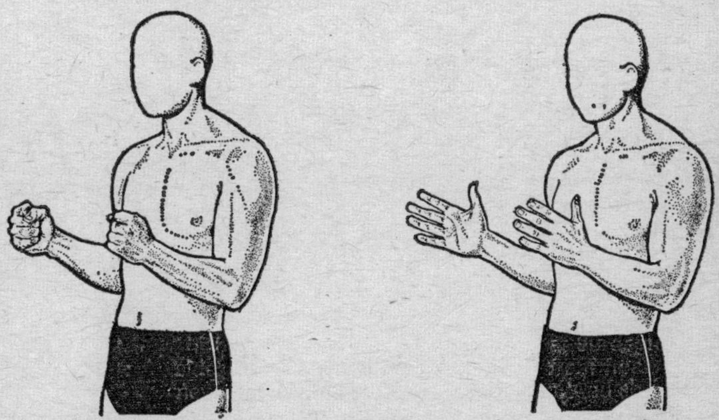

Just ball up fingers and extend them every day. 25 reps a time.

down with the knuckles of the first and second fingers (wrist/ back of your hand should be in a straight line). Can be used on any part of the body, but from a nonpractised expert is often of small effect.

Go it with karate locals (with shuto-uchi/koshi/ippon-ken-zuki).

TOUGHEN THEM EVERY DAY

Make punchplank (as shown) to toughen knuckle skin. Stop hand glancing-off with practice. Focus punch on point 2 in. other side of plank. 100 reps each hand. Foam rubber makes fist pad.

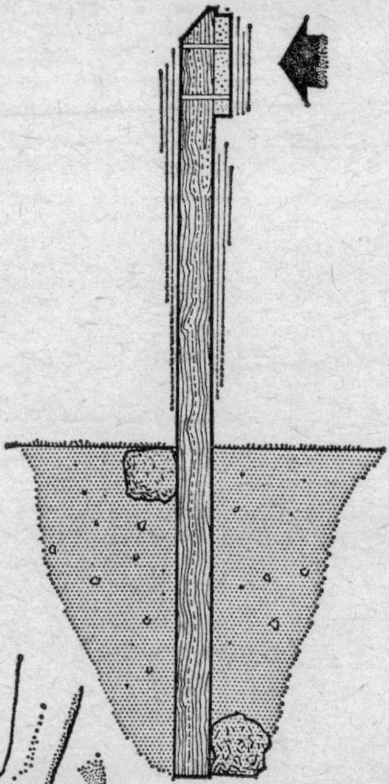

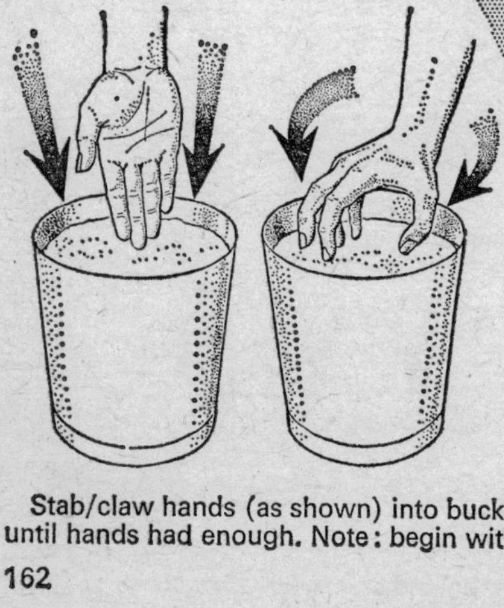

Stab/claw hands (as shown) into bucket of sand/gravel. Reps until hands had enough. Note: begin with bucket of beans.

Squash down 10 fingertips on table to etch fingerprints. Do daily in 6 second sessions.

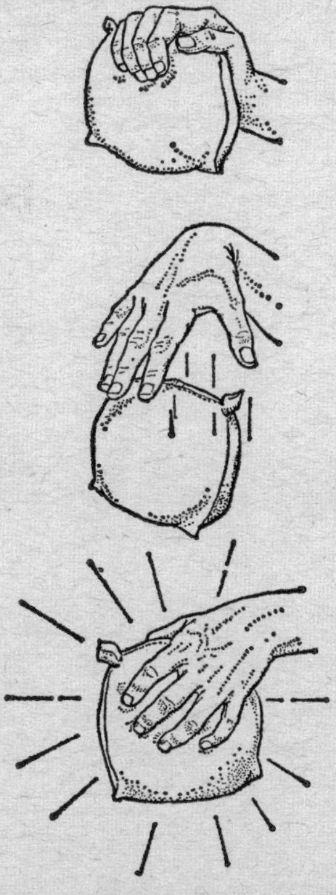

Carry small sand bag (as shown). Drop it and catch from ALL angles with tight finger grab.

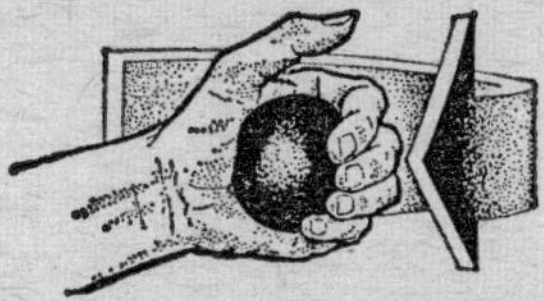

S-q-e-e-e-z-e empty rubber ball in fist 10 reps a time through day.
Crush solid rubber ball (or golf ball) in 6 second efforts.

Screw up DAILY MIRROR middle page at one corner feeding it one-handed into palm until tight ball in fist-that-feels-it.
Then—
Put DAILY MIRROR ball in centre of DAILY TELEGRAPH middle page. Hold with *other* hand. Ball up whole issue into paper sphere one-handed.
Swap sequence around for hands.

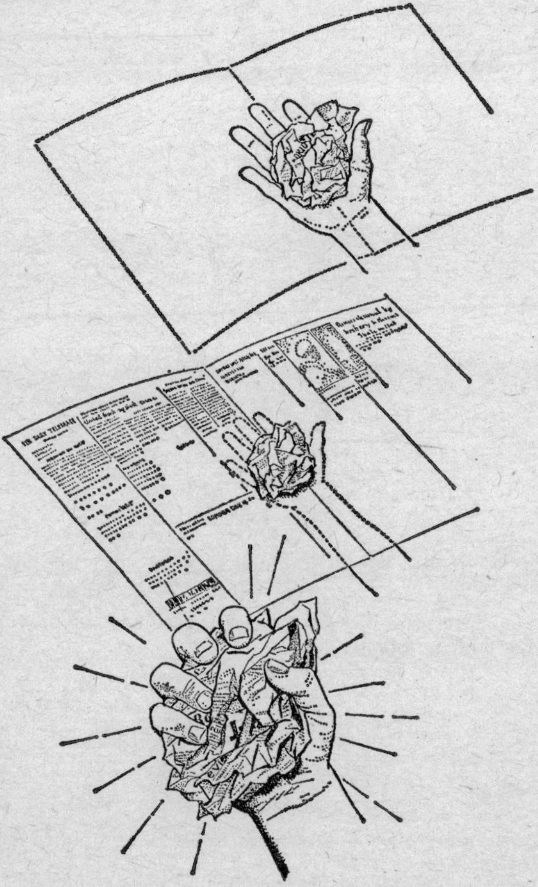

POWER PROGRAMME

Power stuff for those MON/WED/FRI workouts.

IF doing allround bodyplan 3 sets of one of these = enough for 1 night. But if grip rips *nothing* pick 2–3 fist toners (several sets each workout). Wrists*/forearms take loads of stick.

*= measure wrists just above projecting bones NOT round them. Clasp of wristwatch strap/bracelet/band = sure sign muscles growing.

Wrist roller*

Make from 16 in. broomstick pole, 3 foot cord, old electric iron (or scrap). Add weight as you WANT.

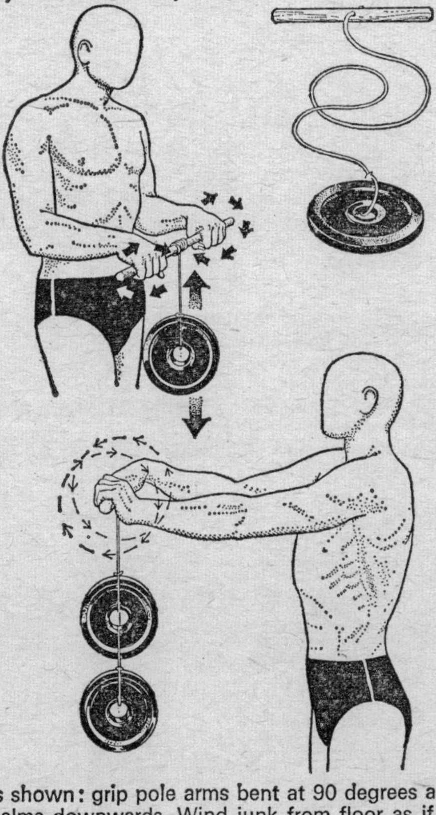

Do as shown: grip pole arms bent at 90 degrees and held to sides, palms downwards. Wind junk from floor as if rolling up newspaper. Winch down to floor again. And so on until tired.

*= WRIST is *some* guide to bodygrowth potential. Mature wrist less than 7 in. = will be tough to gain *massive* physique. But mature wrists in 7½ in.–8 in. class = Muscle Beach body potential. Always exceptions.

ALSO. Do as shown on preceding page, winding weight up *and* DOWN.

Pincer gripping

Makes YOU handshake-king.

Do as shown with single weight discs* or no. of discs centrally loaded on dumbell rod. Pinch weight between thumb-fingers and lift off floor.

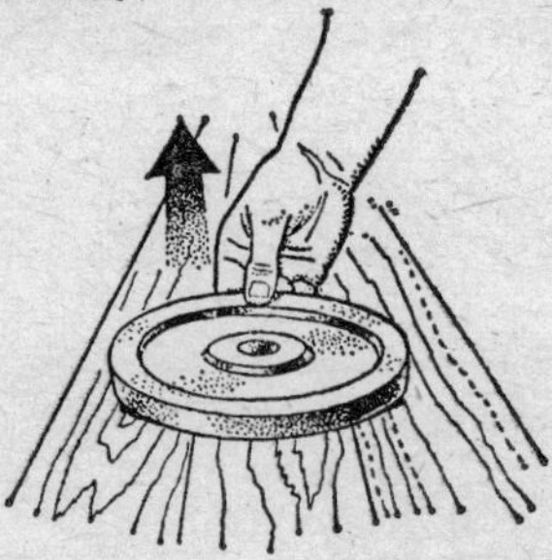

Increase weight until newfound power amazes you. Also toss weight from hand to hand fielding it with pinch grip.

*= or any old iron.

Keeping adding to it.

Ultimate in pinch gripping = THE brick test. *Soon* possible for most men.

Challenge strong man to lift 24 building bricks off ground in one go with one hand in pocket.

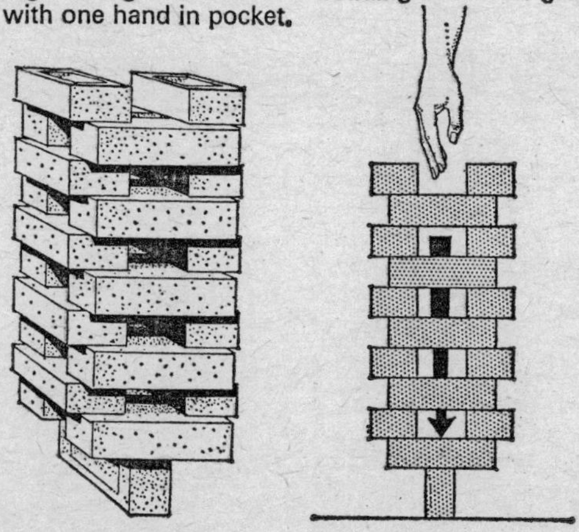

Solution as shown. Brick tower built on foundation brick allows arm to slot right down and hoist that bottom brick with pincer power. Try with fewer bricks first.

Chinning bar

(See BACK.)

But grasp bar with fingers only (NOT fists).

Leverage bell toner

As shown.

Make leverage bell clamping a disc to one end of dumbell rod with 2 collars. Further from disc you grip rod greater resistance to muscles.

Rotate bell. Move up/down. From side to side.

Note: old iron can be improvised into leverage bell shape (like an axe). Pick weight to suit you.

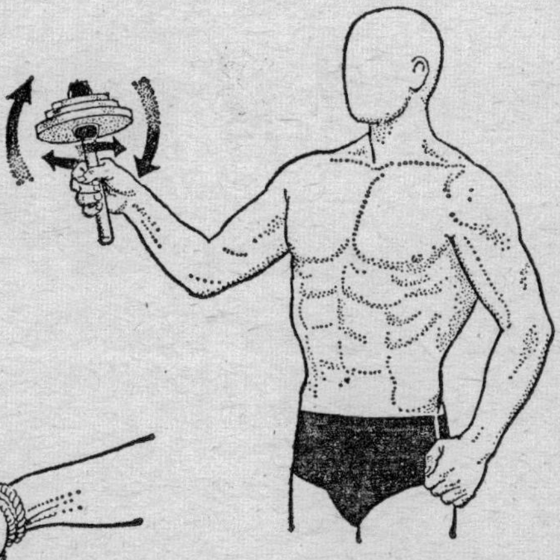

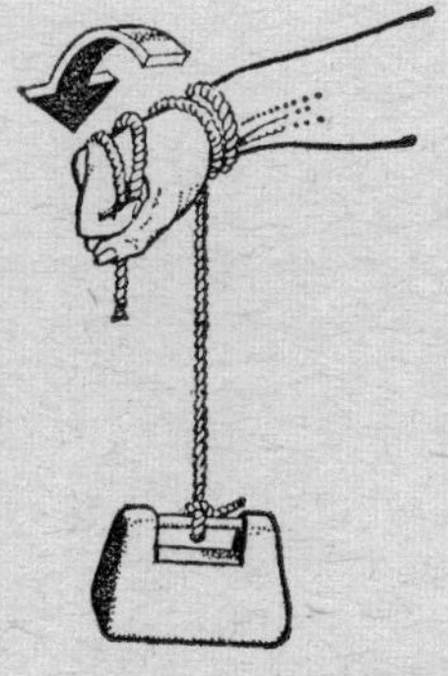

Try this s-l-o-w-l-y

Wrist curl

As shown.

Sit on stool, rest forearms along thighs with hands gripping barbell so fists PROJECT beyond knees. Lift/lower bar by hand movement alone.

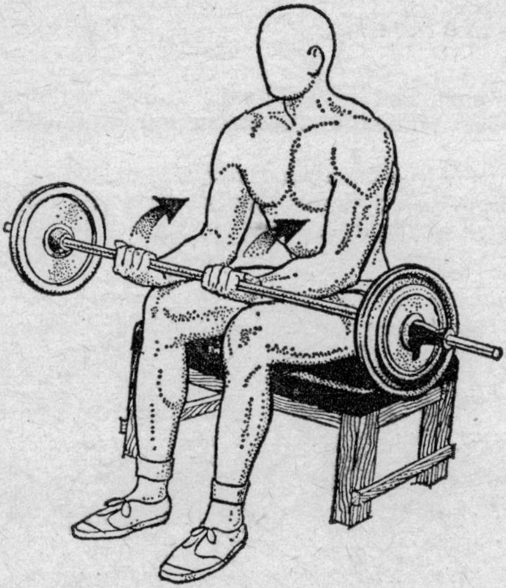

ARMS

ARMS:* 7

**= Upper arms (forearms: see FINGERS/HANDS/WRISTS).*

YOUR ARMS boast Showman's muscle with proper rehearsal (a sideshow flop without). Biceps as big as coconuts only come from hurling them long/hard/zestfully at targets well within YOUR range and present POWer.

Rollup/Rollup/Rollup shirtsleeves to show 18 in. biceps and YOU can have an instant audience. BUT never expect INSTANT success. There are 4 Silver Secrets if you aim to become the world's first 21 in. biceps prize owner.

(1) Slave labour, (2) Variety Bill of exercises NOT just one or two, (3) Torso conditioned by full exercise programme NOT simply *all* slog on arms, (4) Progressive coaxing according to build.

WHAT YOUR ARMS CAN DO TO-DAY

Look good.

Show YOURSELF muscle potential

Clench fist in trad posture of flexing biceps. Press bicep into chest. NOW aim for *that* musclesize with hard packed muscle fibres when arm is held AWAY from body.

Bend 6 in. nails barefisted

(See also FINGERS/HANDS/WRISTS.)

Average strong man can bend them NOW. If doubtful TRY

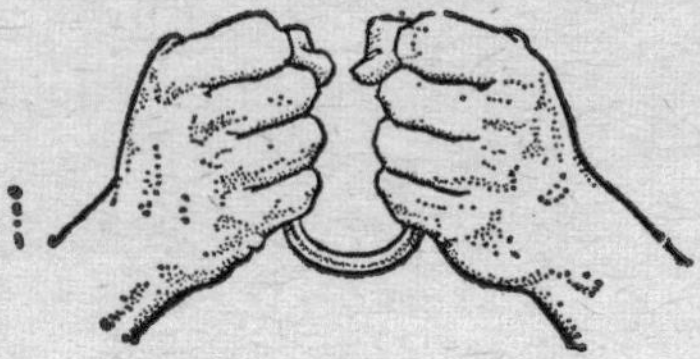

gauge-10 nails (thinner than usual). Work up to thicker gauge thickness.

Practice first.

1. WRAP EACH NAIL END WITH BIT OF CLOTH.
2. GRASP PADS THUS FORMED, EACH PALM FACING UP.
3. GRIP FISTS NEAR CHEST AND ...
4. PRESSURE NAIL STEADILY UPWARDS/INWARDS.
5. NAIL WILL BEND.

Practice first in finding *right grip*. Fail now but keep trying = YOU will do it.

Win at arm wrestling

Take on allcomers after practice. 14 in. arm man licked 20 in. arm opponent in World Arm Wrestling Championships, USA, 1967. Fancy YOUR chances?

WAWC Rules =

(a) Right fist wrestling only.

(b) Thumbs only grip (palms locked at thumbs) as shown.

(c) Ref says READY/GO.

(d) Elbow lifting off table = FOUL. 2 fouls in a match. give pin to opponent.

(e) PROPER PIN = when either battler's hand is *pinned* by opponent's forearm to table. And this wins the match.

TRY to pin/staple/nail protagonist's fist to table by—

1. IMMEDIATELY TRYING TO TWIST OPPONENT'S HAND SO ...
2. YOUR OWN PALM FACES YOUR OWN CHEST.
3. NOW EMPLOY BICEP POWER PLUS FIST FORCE TO ...
4. CURL HIS ARM TOWARDS YOU WITH DOWN-COILING PRESSURE.

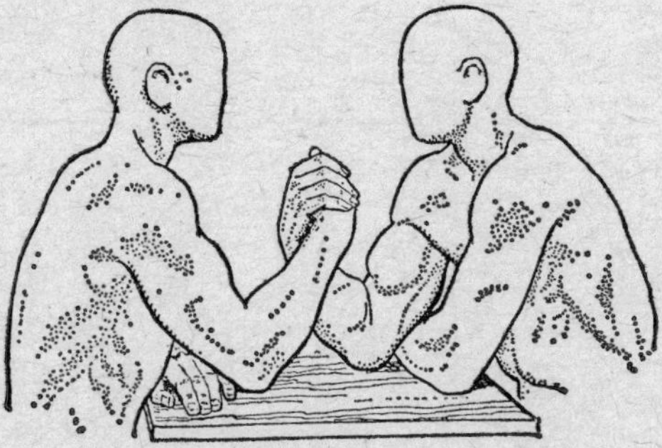

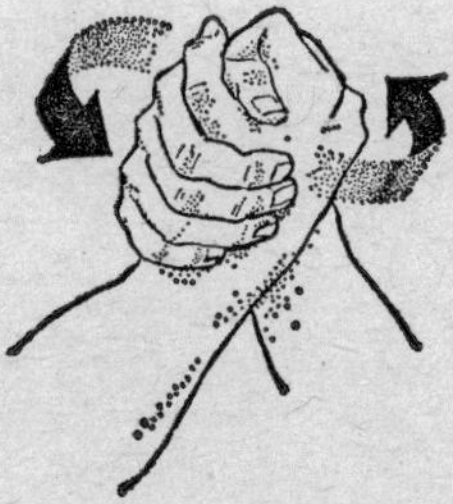

5. NEXT TRY TO BEND YOUR FIST TO YOUR WRIST AND . . .
6. BRING IN SHOULDER POWER BY FORCING IT FORWARD TO AID THAT ARM.
7. PRESS/PRESS/PRESS ON TABLE WITH FREE HAND.
8. AND FORCE HIS HAND FLAT ON TABLE.

One-handed pullups
As shown overleaf.

THE acme of manly strength. So many utterly fail this powertest. Start PRACTISING to-day.

Grow strong from arm exercises. And the knack can be practised.

1. GRIP BAR WITH BOTH HANDS (PALMS IN) AND PULLUP
2. HOLD ON FOR A MOMENT WITH CHIN ABOVE IT.
3. LET GO WITH WEAKEST HAND.

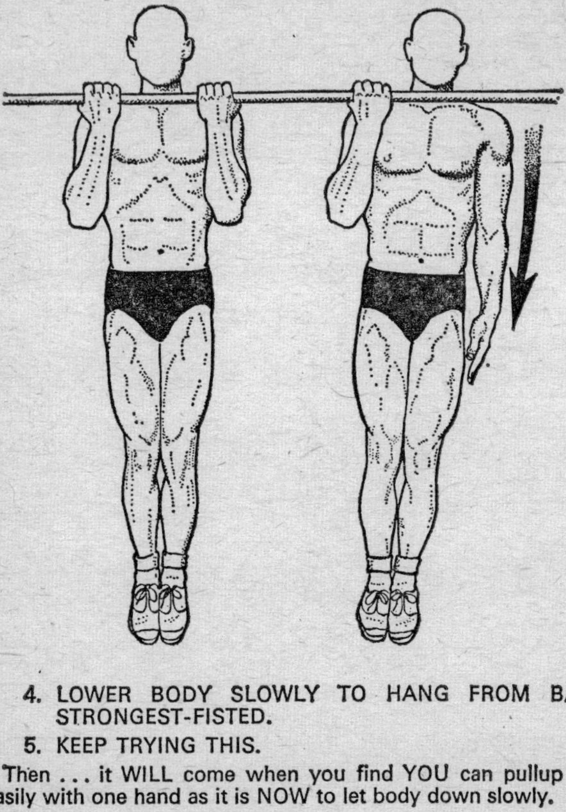

4. LOWER BODY SLOWLY TO HANG FROM BAR STRONGEST-FISTED.
5. KEEP TRYING THIS.

Then . . . it WILL come when you find YOU can pullup as easily with one hand as it is NOW to let body down slowly.

PACK ARM LIMBERING DAILY

Unusual IF those arms well developed now (few are to-day). Arms often thin/puny/stringy, Biceps/triceps need driving. Gearup to-day if painfully weak.

Pick selection of arm limberers. Swap around as you need to cover ALL exercises (again, if weak). BUT don't chop/change over a few days trial.
(See also ABDOMEN; CHEST/SHOULDERS/BACK; BODY.)

Good pushups

(See also SHOULDERS.)

Go prone with toes curled under, handpalms in line with

shoulders, fingers pointing forwards. Take normal breath. Push body from floor until arms straight. Lower body to start (blowing-out on waydown).
Note: in UP position body is deadstraight with weight on toes/hands. TRY if hard at first. 25 reps = excellent progress.

Vertical pressups

As shown.

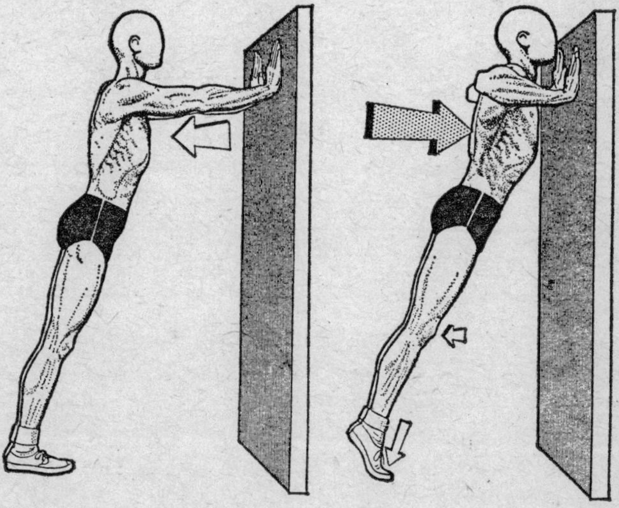

Very easy. But pile on reps (rising on toes/pushing hard/giving all).

Arm stretcher

(*See also FINGERS/HANDS/WRISTS.*)

Hold broom handle above/behind head. Twist one fist backwards, other forward at same time pulling out at sides along length of handle. Just feel arm muscles stretching and aching after 60 seconds (tyro's limit).
Note: arms should = 90 degrees bend.

Pumper

(*See also CHEST.*)

Pump arms back/forth with vim. Fists clenched/knuckles pointing IN one time/OUT next.

Chair dips
As shown.

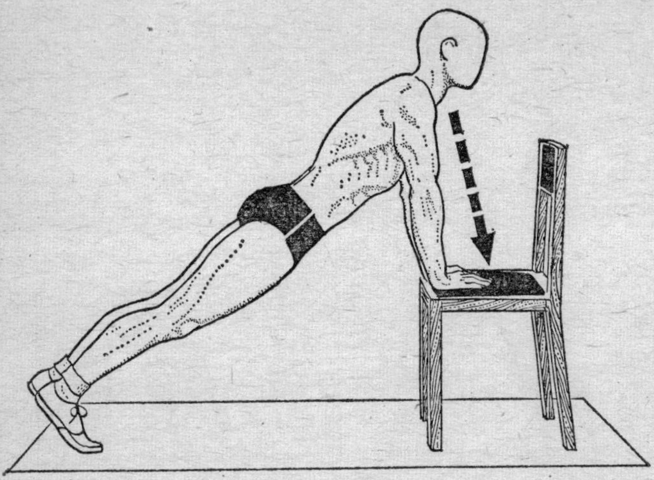

1. GRASP CHAIR SEAT EDGE UNDER HANDHEELS.
2. POSITION FEET ON NONSLIP FLOOR SO...
3. BODY IS STRAIGHT.
4. LOWER FACE TO CHAIR WITH ELBOWS AT 90 DEGREES TO BODY.
5. PUSH ON HANDS SLOWLY JACKING UP BODY UNTIL...
6. ARMS ARE STRAIGHT (AND BODY RIGID).

Start with 10 reps. Work up to 20.

Tugger
As shown.

Use teatowel wrapped round fist. Yank free end with other. Hard/hard/hard to make muscles slog.

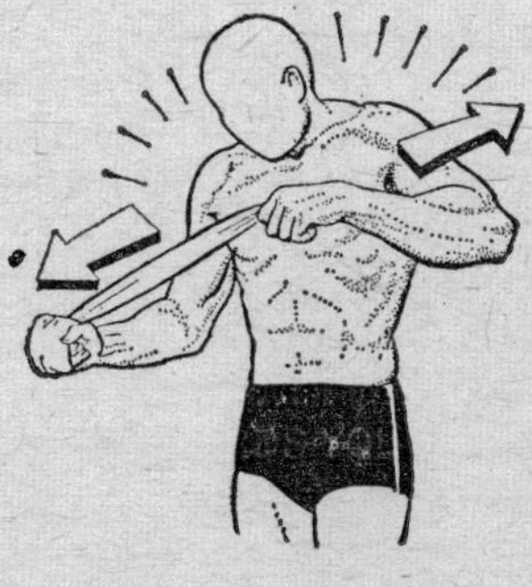

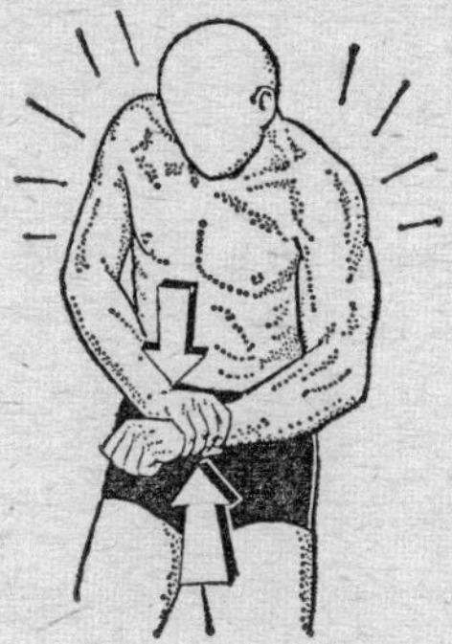

Presser

As shown.

Keep up pressure of one fist on other wrist to blowup biceps/triceps.

Chinning

As shown.

Do it anywhere/anytime/anyhow (with knuckles pointing both OUT and IN. Use low branches/door lintels/oak beams. Use body weight = resistance for triceps/biceps.

INSTANT MICROMOVERS

Universal tensioners OK for ANY place. Do them daily. 6 seconds a shot.

Arm contraction

Stand straight with left fist in right palm (forearms parallel to floor). Take deep breath and TRY to raise RIGHT palm while fightback with LEFT (6 seconds).

Then swap.

Pressing-down contraction

Reverse of above.

Stand with right fist cupped in left palm (left arm brought across body). Breathe in and press down HARD with right fist (being checked by left hand). 6 second swaps.

Handclasp shoving

As shown overleaf.

Mince palms together (prayer position). Breathe in and crush for 6 seconds.

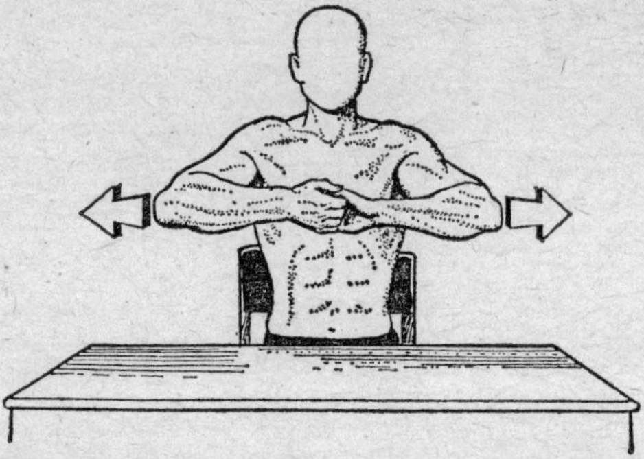

Handclasp ripping

As shown.

With elbows out at sides/arms parallel to floor/deep breath. Order brain: RIVE HANDS APART. But don't let it. 6 seconds battle. Try opposite for 6.

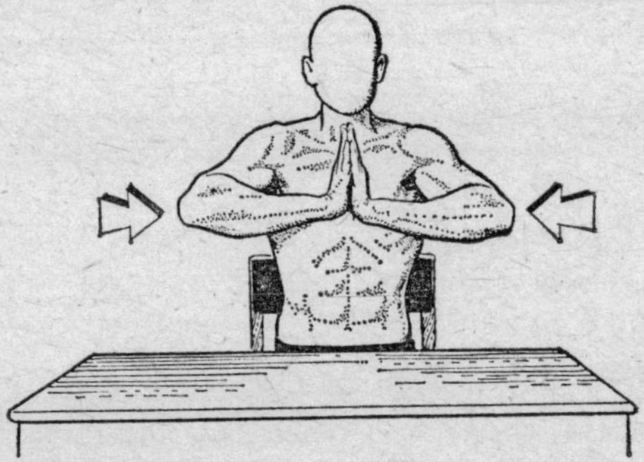

Hand ripping behind head

Link fingers at necknape. Try to divorce with 6 seconds strife.

Neck spoiler

Grip right fist in left palm. Bring grasp overhead to headback SO right biceps nudge right ear. Standup. And breathin. TRY to rocket RIGHT FIST overhead but halt with other hand. 6 seconds countdown.

Tabletop pressdown

Sit close to table palms on top (at shoulder width/elbows tucked to sides/arms bent at 90 degrees). Adjust height for this with stool/chair/cushion. 6 mad seconds pressure.

Widegrip desk squeezer

As shown (both ways).

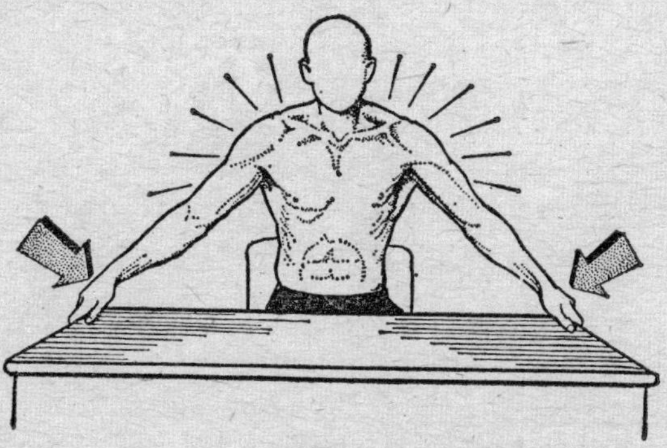

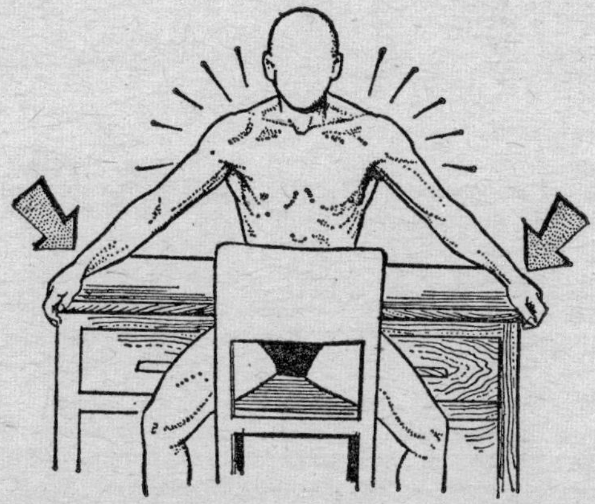

DO both ways. Keeping back straight/eyes ahead/feeling power rays spurting out of YOU. Use 6 seconds pressure infront/behind.

Undergrip

At desk/sink/carbumper grip UNDER rim bothhanded. TRY to raise palms + object into sky. For 6 seconds. By bending elbows.

Desk leaner

As shown overleaf.

Body straight/heels of hands pushing/looking ahead. Aim eyeballs for 6 seconds ramdown FORCE on desk.

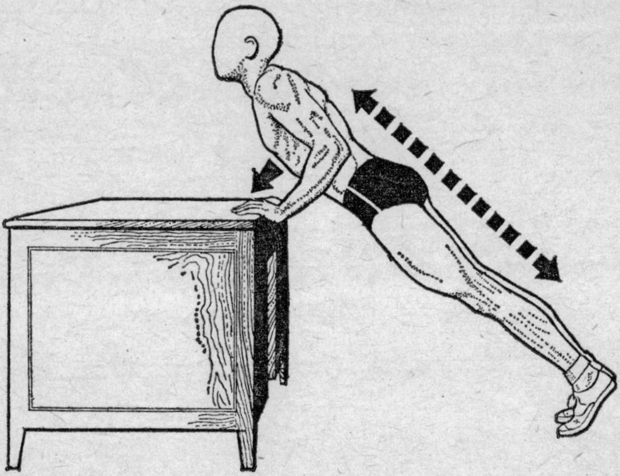

Back wall push

Stand 15 in. from wall (behind you). Have arms by sides, palms facing wall. Keep arms straight. PRESS on wall like madman for 6 (eyes ahead/back straight/chestfull).

Doorway pusher

Stand in doorway centre. Raise arms. Reach out/out/out. Both palms checked by jambs. Go for 6 seconds door pushdown.

Towel spoiler

Sit/stand. Stretch folded towel taut (hands across chest; palms out). Raise elbows sideways. Keep arms parallel with floor. Breathe in. TRY to shear towel apart for 6 seconds.

Towel tugging

Floorsit legs out together. Pass towel round insteps gripping with both arms straightout. Reach forward roundbacked.

Breathein/tossback head/tugback for 6 blinding seconds. Push/pull with legs/arms.

Towel curl

As shown opposite.

Lock towel under right foot. Grip other end with righthand (about waist height). Yank towel taut arm flexed at 90 degrees (elbow glued to side). TRY *full arm flexing* on breath-in. Do 6 second swaps.

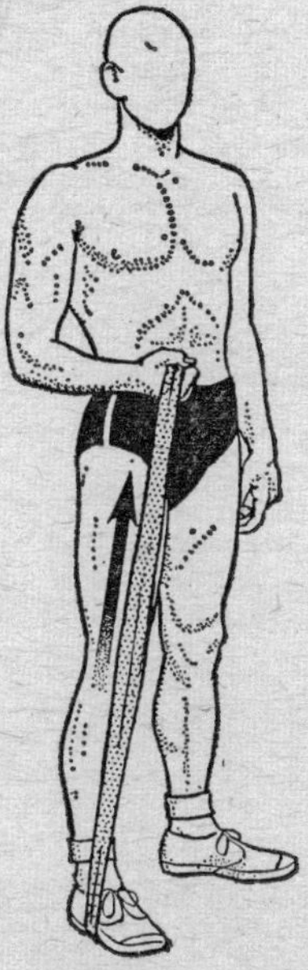

UPPER ARM POWER PRODUCING

THE programme.

Tapemeasure (1) straightout arm at shoulder level with muscle relaxed and at thickest point. *And* (2) around fully flexed bicep.

Best test = bicepscrammed suitsleeves.

Workover arms with BIG exercise range. *Remember.*

FOR weightgaining = at least 1 tricep *and* 1 bicep powerpacker in MON/WED/FRI routine using maximum weights (3 sets of 10 reps).

FOR powergaining = use 2 tricep *and* 2 bicep exercises in programme (4–5 sets of 6 reps).

FOR fitnessgaining = at least 1 tricep *and* 1 bicep fitnessfixer (3 sets of 15–20 reps).

Swap exercises at 6–8 week periods. Tryout new for next 2 weeks. Then begin NEW 6–8 week session. And attack muscles from NEW angles. Change at least half original exercise programme. Powerpackers you DON'T drop from original session must be dropped for 3rd 6–8 week's period. You can always bring them back for later 6–8 weekly sessions.

YOU must shock stubborn muscle into growth. Try NEW angle approach when stuck. Hit muscle with allround ex.

Note: keep to same *order* of body parts each 6–8 week's period: e.g. legs first; then chest/shoulders/back; then arms, etc.

VITAL: to bomb/blitz/shell biceps AND triceps with dual-direction exercise.

BICEPS

NEVER use barbells *only*. Dumbell powerers give VARIETY.

Barbell curl

As shown.

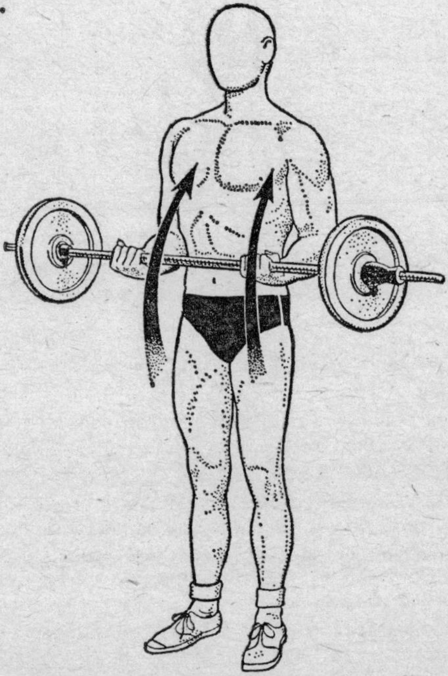

1. STAND FEET APART, BARBELL HANGING ACROSS THIGHS.
2. AND PALMS FACING FRONTWAYS.
3. CURL BAR TO UPPER CHEST/NECK BY ...
4. BENDING ARMS SMOOTHLY.

5. LOWER AND REPEAT.

Note: upper arm muscles DO work. NOT bodyswing *nor* shouldershrug. Use arms only for POWer. Hand spacing = shoulder width. Keep elbows from body on UP.

Alternate dumbell curl

As shown.

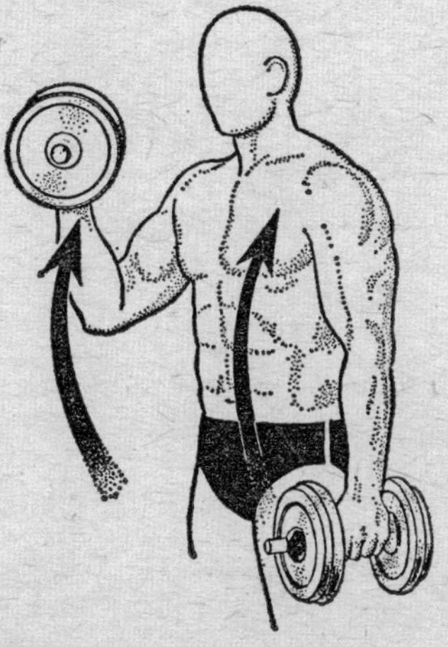

1. STAND FEET APART HOLDING DUMBELLS AT HANG POSITION.
2. PALMS FACING IN.
3. CURL ONE BELL TO SHOULDER ...
4. TURNING PALM UPPERMOST.
5. LOWER BELL AND CURL WITH OTHER.

Keep swapping bells until enough reps done.
Note: expect to use less weight than with barbell.

Seated swingbell curl

As shown overleaf.

Swingbell = centrally loaded dumbell rod. NOT too heavy: no body motion allowed to help.

1. SIT ON LOW STOOL ...
2. LEGS APART/KNEES BENT/SWINGBELL NEAR FLOOR.
3. KNUCKLES DOWN/ARMS STRETCHED/ELBOWS ON INNER THIGHS.

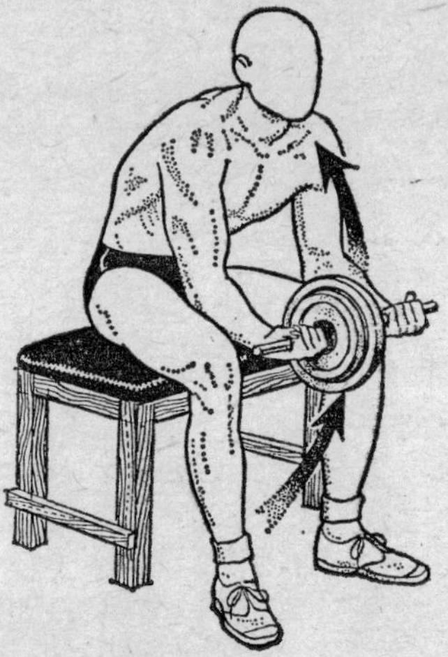

4. AND GIVE IT HELL ...
5. BY CURLING UP SWINGBELL UNTIL CHEST/NECK TOUCHED.

3 sets of 10 reps.

Note: no body movement at all = RIGHT way. Strict movement = RIGHT way. NO wrist bendover = RIGHT way. Muscle afterburn = RIGHT way.

Concentration curl

As shown opposite.

1. SIT ON BENCH EDGE HOLDING DUMBELL RIGHT-HANDED.
2. AND LET ARM PLUMBLINE DOWN BETWEEN KNEES (KNUCKLES FORWARD).
3. LEAN BODY FORWARD AND ...
4. HAVE NONLIFTING HAND AS SHOWN.
5. FREEZE BODY BUT RAISE DUMBELL TO RIGHT SHOULDER BY ...
6. FULLY BENDING ARM ...
7. TURNING FIST INWARDS AS IT IS RAISED.
8. RETURN DUMBELL TO START TWISTING HAND OUT.

3 sets of 8 reps an arm.
Biceps ache = natural.

Note: heavy dumbells *out* in this special toneup. Weight is NOT object. Great concentration and deliberation IS. NEVER swing

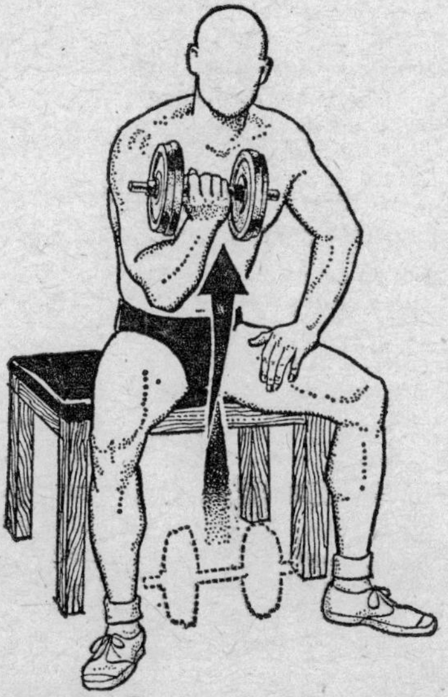

bell up. Use poundage that just allows 8–12 reps. And CURL it.

Across chest curl
As shown. (Described overleaf.)

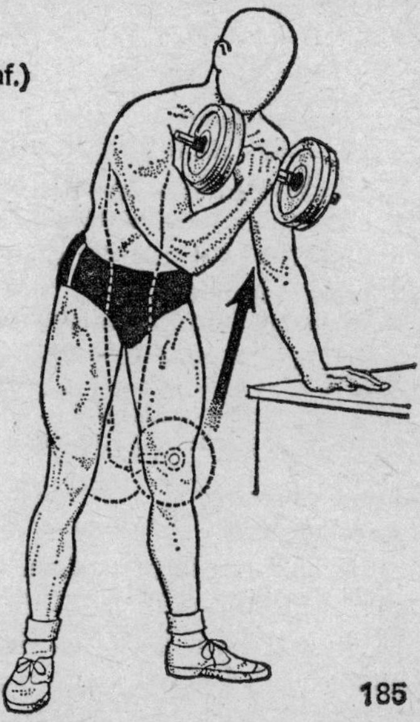

1. STAND LEANING FORWARD FROM WAIST AND PRESS ...
2. FREE HAND ON BENCH/TABLE/STOOL WHILE ...
3. OTHER ARM HANGS STRAIGHT WITH DUMBELL.
4. KEEP UPPER ARM FROZEN AND BEND FOREARM + BELL ...
5. SO IT CROSSES CHEST TO OPPOSITE SHOULDER.
6. PAUSE BRIEFLY AND LOWER TO START.

3 sets of 8 reps an arm.
Note: NEVER sway body.

Prone bench curl

As shown.

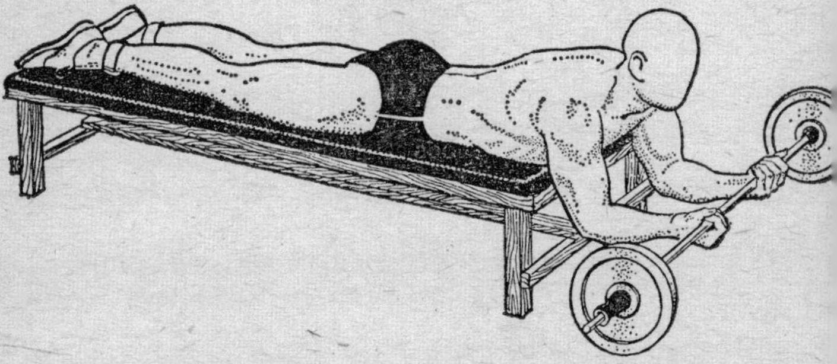

1. LIE PRONE ON TRAINING BENCH WITH ...
2. SHOULDERS/ARMS JUTTING OVER END.
3. GRASP BARBELL THEN ...
4. FULLY BEND ARMS RAISING IT TO SHOULDERS.
5. LOWER IT UNDER CONTROL.

3 sets of 10 reps.
Note: do NOT floortouch bar between reps.

TRICEPS

Armback muscle = ENEMY to biceps. Give triceps share of clog or THEY clogup whole arm movement (see BODY).

French press

As shown.

Can be done sitting/standing.

1. HOLD BARBELL ABOVE HEAD (HANDS 6 in. APART).
2. LOWER BAR TO NECKNAPE KEEPING ELBOWS HIGH.

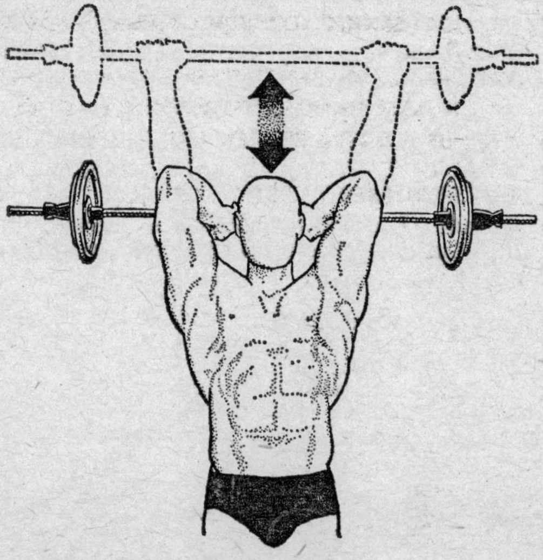

3. AND PRESS BACK UP TO ARMS OUT POSITION.
4. KEEP IT UP.

Note: use as little help as possible from UPPER arm movement. Until arms locked straight elbows ALWAYS point to roof.

Single arm triceps stretch

As shown. Described overleaf

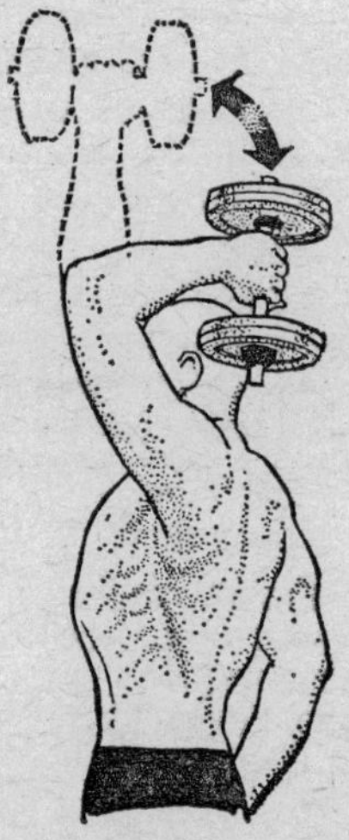

A variant on above exercise.

1. GRIP DUMBELL AT ARM'S LENGTH OVERHEAD AND ...
2. LOWER BELL TO NECKNAPE WHILE ...
3. KEEPING ELBOW HIGH/BICEPS TOUCHING SKULL.
4. PRESS BELL OVERHEAD WITH MINIMUM UPPER ARM MOVEMENT.

Note: sit/stand; concentrate/concentrate/concentrate; once elbow DROPS muscle value LOST; fold free arm across chest out of way.

Lying barbell triceps stretch

As shown.

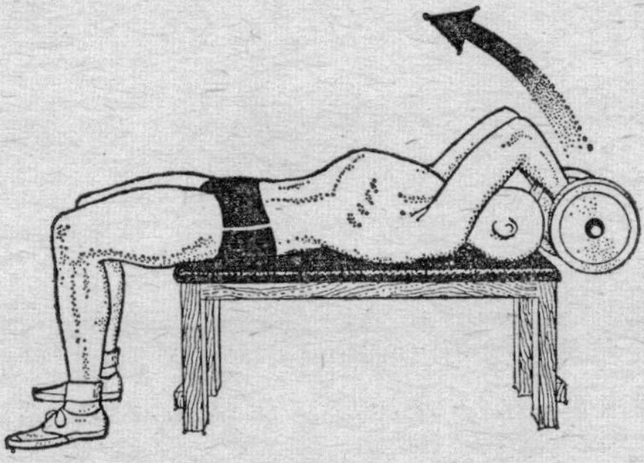

1. LIE ON BENCH LOOKING UP AND ...
2. BARBELL AT FULL ARMS OUT OVER FACE (6 in. ARM SPACING).
3. LOWER BAR UNTIL DROPPING JUST BEHIND HEAD.
4. PRESS BACK OVER FACE.
5. LOWER AND REPEAT.

Note: keep upper arms statuesque during motions. THOUGH some movement up here—cut it to minimum. Just allow enough to allow bar to clear head on way down.

Tricep dips

As shown.

(See also SHOULDERS/BACK.)

Use horizontal bars or 2 strong chair backs (need to knees-bend here on descent movement).

1. TAKE SUPPORT POSITION AS SHOWN.

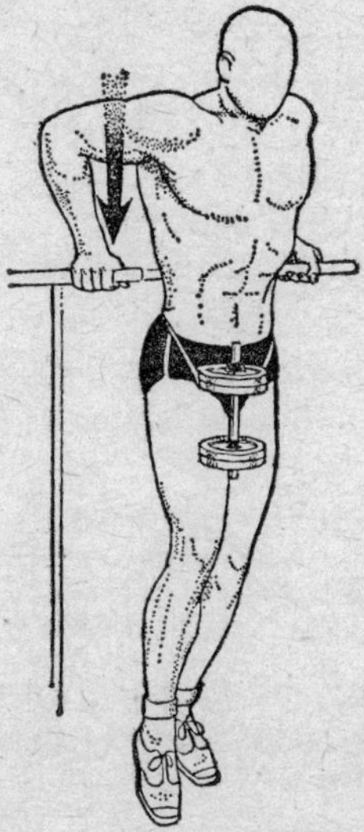

2. LOWER/RAISE BODY BY BENDING/STRETCHING ARMS SO . . .
3. YOU ENSURE GOOD LOCKOUT AT ARMS STRETCH.

Breathe in on lowering; out on raising. When too easy tie discs/old iron/junk to waist to = added resistance.

Triceps lever

Make up weighted disc on dumbell rod (as shown). Or make

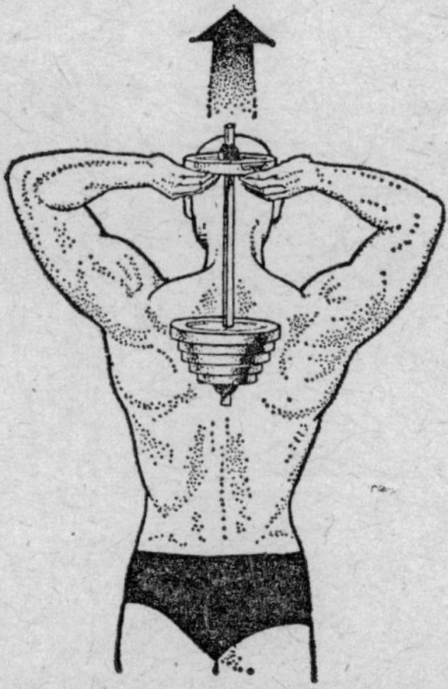

weight of old electric kettle sandfilled, etc.

1. SLIP FINGERS UNDER WEIGHT AND ...
2. PRESS TO FULL ARMS STRETCH OVERHEAD.
3. LOWER WEIGHT TO WELL BEHIND HEAD ...
4. FULLY BENDING ELBOWS.
5. STEADILY STRAIGHTEN ARMS LOCKING ELBOWS FOR BEST CONTRACTION.

3 sets of 10 reps.

Note: upper arms MUST remain still—elbows jabbing high. Check collars of dumbell so weights safe.

Rear triceps extension

Grip dumbell onehanded. Other hand presses low bench, etc. Extend weighted arm backwards until FULLY locked. Pause. Return to start. Skip worries about lack of poundage = makes this possible. So long as triceps ache after: POWer.

READYFOUND POWER GEAR ADDITIONS

Slot all/any of these into power programme (following Iron Game principles above). ALL as shown.

Inner tubing

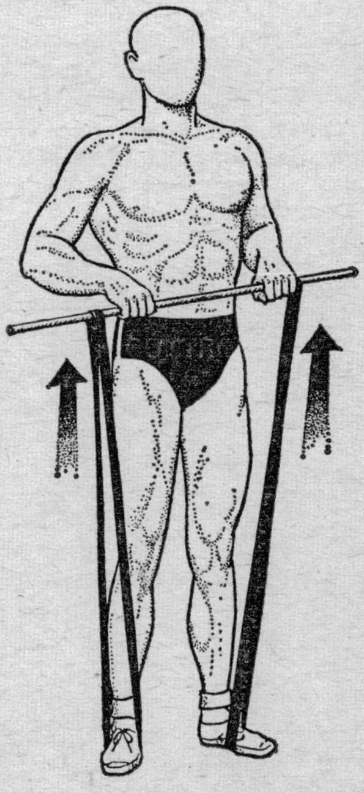

OVERHEAD PRESSES forcing rubber from waistgrip to overhead (feet looped through tubing).

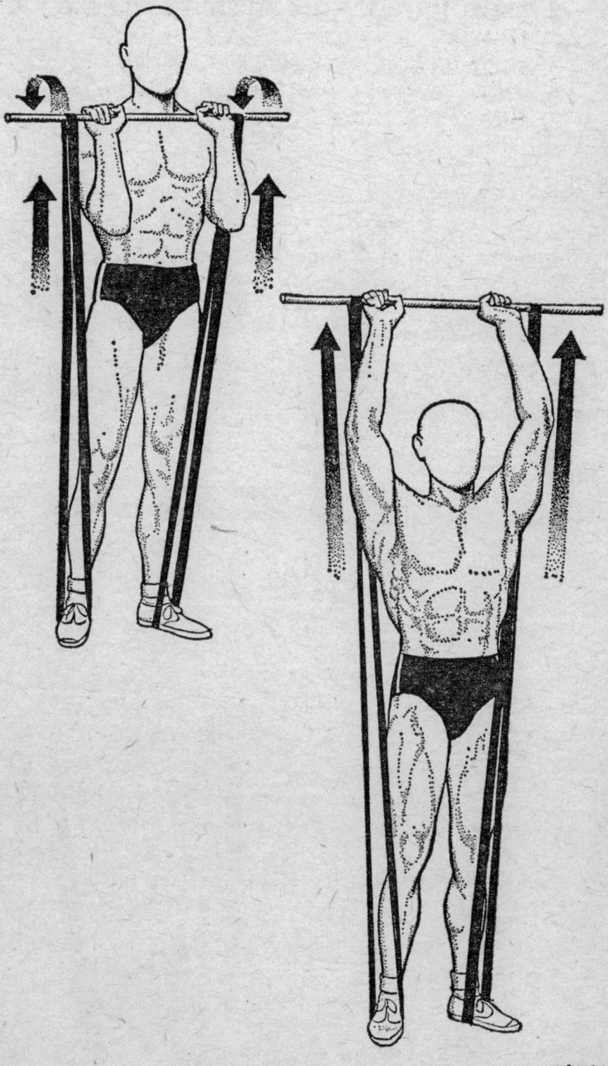

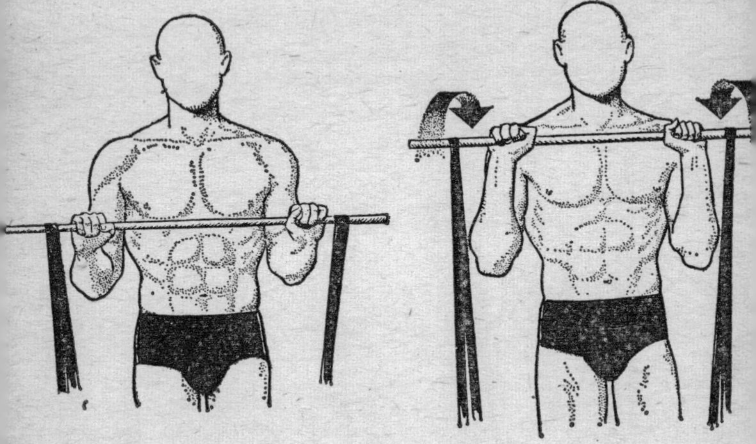

TUBE CURLS as smoothly as with barbell.
REVERSE TUBE CURLS with knuckles pointing OUT.

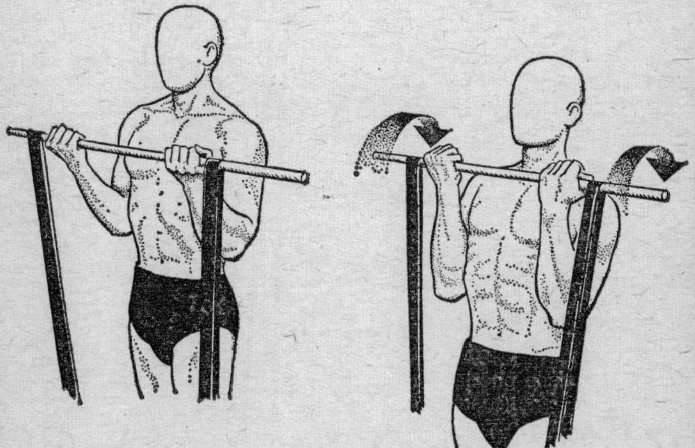

Sandbags

SANDBAG CURLS. As smoothly as with tube curls.

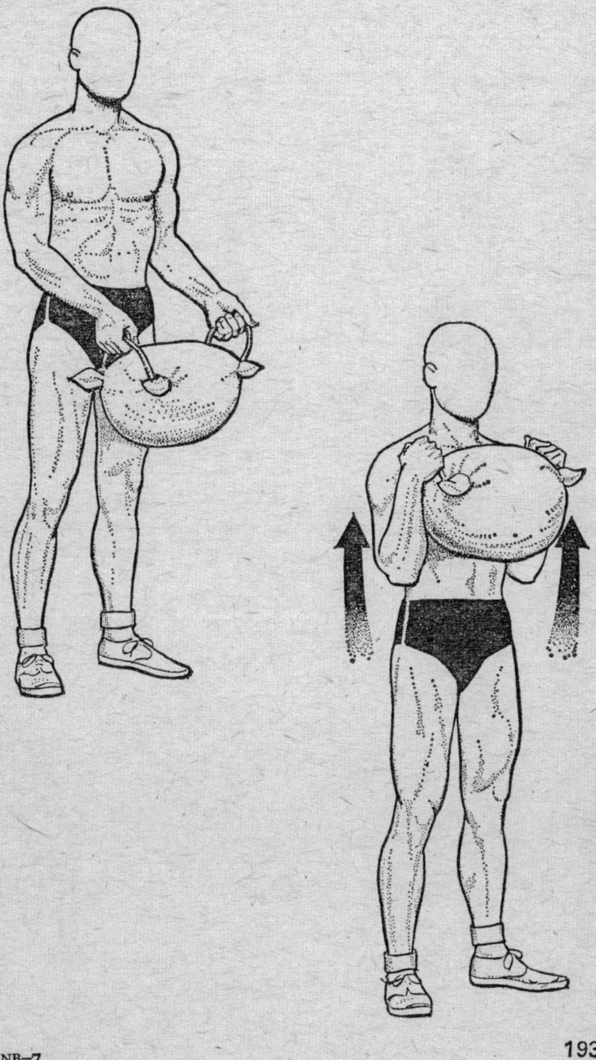

SANDBAG STRAIGHTARM LIFTS from gripping sandbag by thighs to bringing it up to parallel-to-floor position at full arms stretch. And hold there. Lower slowly.

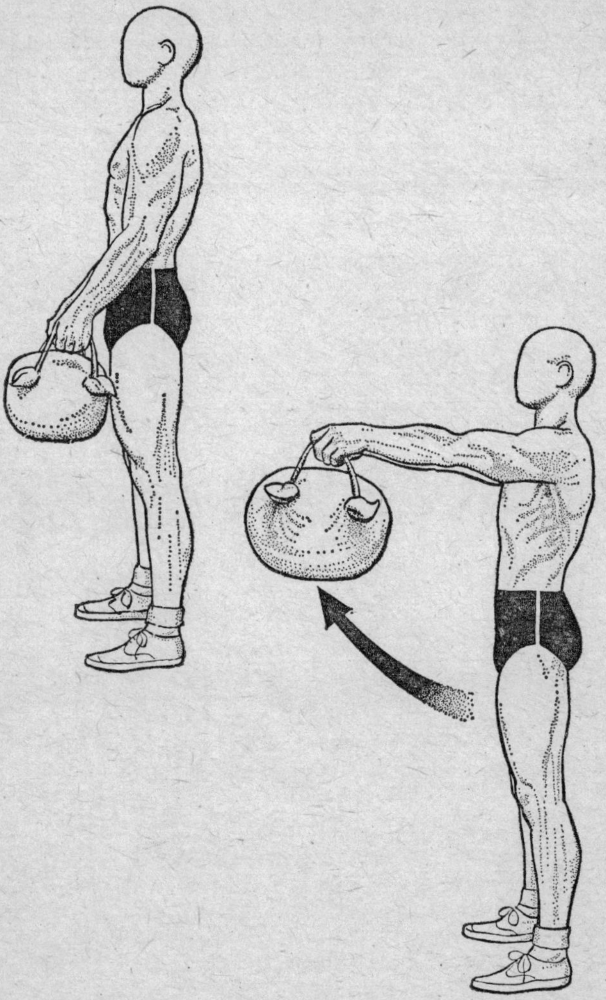

SANDBAG HOISTS by pushing bag up vertically from headtop. And down/up/down, etc.

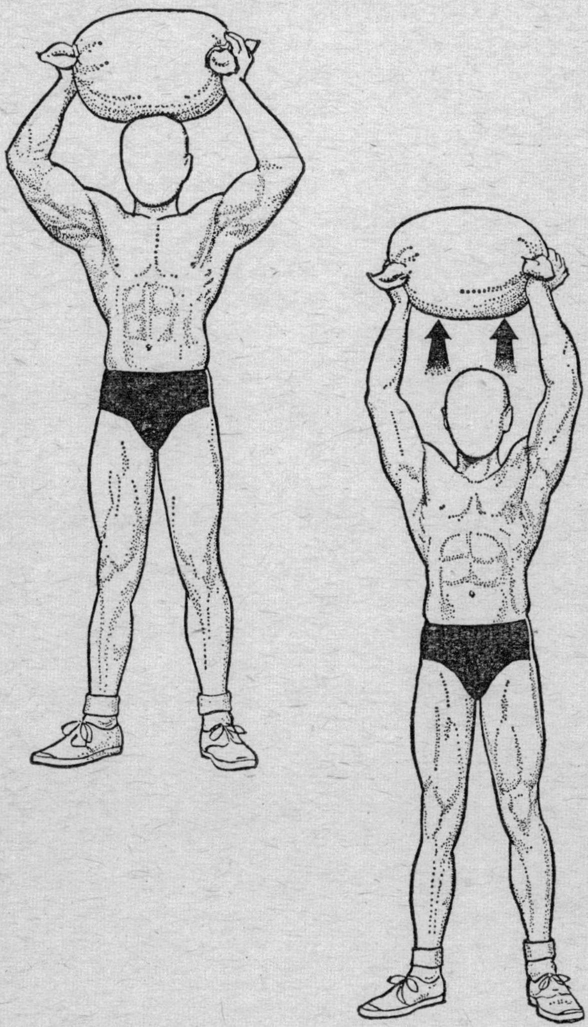

NECK

NECK: 8

YOUR NECK shows YOU as MR TOUGH or MR SOFT at a glance. Logthick column of vibrant power = best barometer of health/strength/vigour whether wearing best suit/denims/ British warm. Unfit, untough: it shows HERE first.

Bullneck IS best survival kit to man. Car crashes/falls/fights ALL cushioned better. 18 in. neck has proved lifesaver buffer when hit by 1 cwt. flour sack crashing 20 feet. An oxneck = tough upper spine.

Is YOUR neck weak/scrawny/emaciated? Have YOU flabby double chins? Let MR TOUGH crane your neck to new heights of chiselled power. Warning: don't buy new shirts for a month (you will soon burst collars).

STICK THAT NECK OUT NOW

With power already inside it.

Hang by neck from 2 chairs
(*See also ABDOMEN.*)
As shown overleaf.
Lie (as shown) between 3 chairs, head on one, heels on other, glutes on another. Clasp hands across stomach. Blow out breath (= contract muscles). Arch spine.

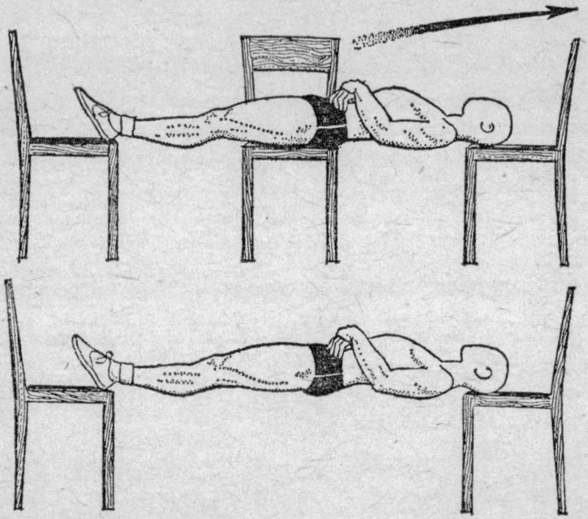

Have middle chair removed.

Neck (and abdomen) will support you rigid for seconds. Fit man takes time to jacknife to floor.

Growing power = set chairs up yourself, take away centre one while lying. And pass it round body to put it under other side of you.

Hoist up a big man with neck power

As shown.

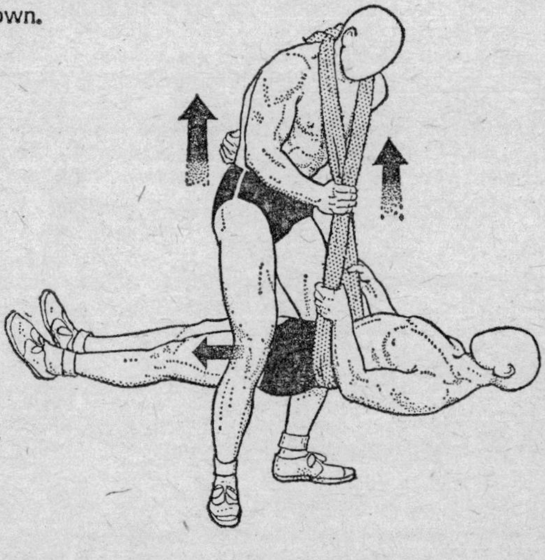

Man lies on floor. Stand by his side. Loop reef-knotted bath towel round his waist and twist into figure of 8. Loop towel top round YOUR neck, bending knees. Plant feet firm. Hold fingers of one hand on towel twist as stabiliser (NOT puller).

1. CONCENTRATE ON LEGS*.
2. PUT ALL EFFORT INTO STRAIGHTENING LEGS.
3. USE NECK SIMPLY AS BRACKET TO LIFT MAN AT LEAST 1 FOOT.

*= *as with LEG-chapter-feat-on-manlifting use legs as power jacks. But neck as powered platform.*

NEVER NEGLECT NECK

Easily ricked—avoid SUDDEN jerks/twists/pulls. Apply any pressure gradually. Also give draughts a miss (like rogue airflo car ventilation) : neck easily cricked.

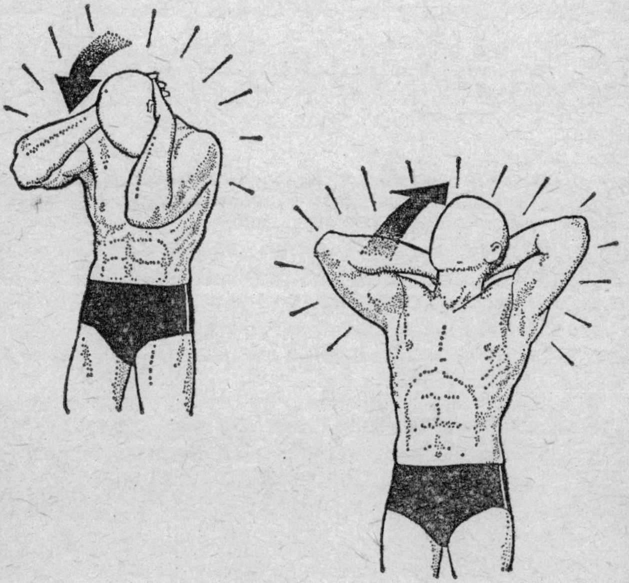

DAILY NECK TOUGHENERS

(a) Clasp hands behind neck. FORCE head back against their unbudging bracelet for 6 seconds.

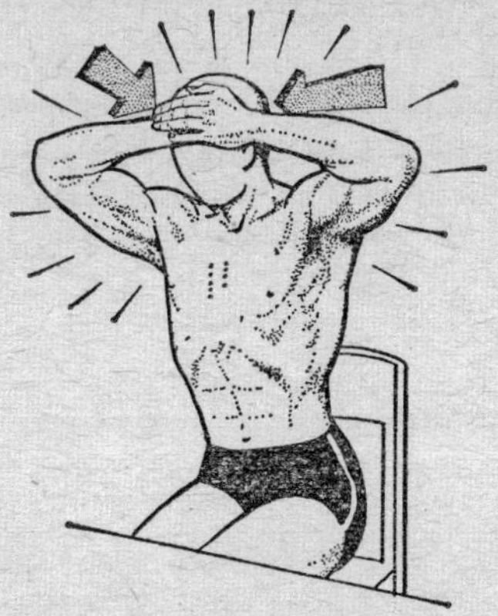

(b) Ram palms to brow, elbows forward. TRY to buffet head forward. But holdfast with hands for 6 seconds.

(c) Slap right hand palm above right ear, elbow out to side. ATTEMPT to turn head right for 6 unbending seconds.

(d) Ditto same as (c) with left hand/left ear/left effort.

(e) Look over left shoulder blade and press right hand palm to right temple. TRY to look *hard* right now against immovable 6 second pressure.

(f) Ditto same as (e) with right gaze/left temple/left effort.

(g) Toss back head cupping chin in hand. Do 6 second skull FORCING onto hand heel.

(h) Drop chin to chest, clasping hands across head crown. These stop up straining skull from reaching chin level (6 seconds).

ALL above exercises toughened by lying on bed/divan/couch with head over the end. Gravity = extra resistance.

(i) Double towel into short hawser. Pull it taut round brow (both hands facing behind skull; elbows raised). TRY to shove head *forward*, towel *backwards* for 6 seconds battle.

(j) Do opposite with back-of-head towel (pull taut both handed). Flex arms at 90 degrees, elbows to front. For 6 seconds straining hands almost touch ears.

(k) Stand in doorway and press brow against jamb (use towel/duster/cloth pad). Lean forward. Balance hands each jamb side. Do BIG 6 second press.

(l) Do opposite with jamb/pad at skull back. Tilt head

back until jamb felt. Hold on to jamb loosehanded behind in 6 second fight.

Note: neck thrives on hard resistance for growth. BUT 3 basic freehand toners are . . .

(m) Roll skull around up/down. Strain against rolling/dipping motion to tone traps/sternomastoid. Reroll.

(n) Lace fingers at skull back and pull arms as you dip head forward/backward. Strong pressure = good muscle.

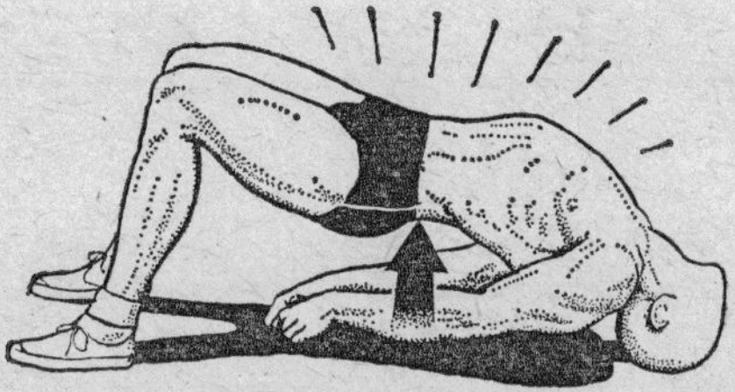

(o) Lie flat on back, draw heels up to glutes and arch body off floor until supported only by head crown*—foot soles. Fold arms across chest. IF you fail due to confidence-lack push with arms besides head thro' first weeks.

Once bridged properly lower body till weight on shoulders. Raise to head top again. 6 reps. Then to 12.

*= *aim to support bridge weight nearer forehead than actual head crown.*

BRIDGE = strong neck. Make exercise even tougher when ready by—

Twisting body from side to side in rocking sway. And adding light weight (like book) on to abs. Try iron-play later.

POWER PRODUCING PROGRAMME

Generally have 1 neck exercise from below in MON/WED/FRI routine. IF neck a wreck 2–3 of these powerpackers will salvage it. In 2–3 sets each.

Up to YOU re poundages/reps for neck. Only use what neck can stand—especially in bridge toners. Aim for plenty reps but NOT too much weight. 3 sets at most.

Neck best measured at slimmest zone just under chin (never across Adam's apple). Burst shirts = best success sign.

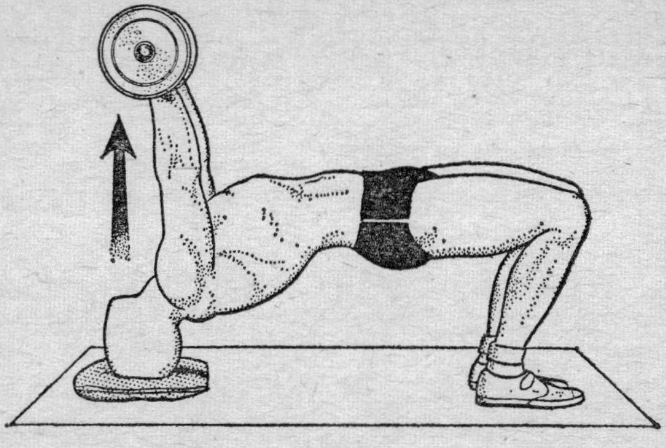

Barbell bridge (Press)

1. ASSUME BRIDGE SPAN POSTURE.
2. HAVE TRAINING MATE HAND YOU LOADED BARBELL AT ARMS' LENGTH OVER CHEST (see CHEST).
3. LOWER BAR TO CHEST AND PRESS BACK UP AT ARMS' STRETCH.
4. DO MORE REPS UNTIL NECK TIRED.

Note: very tough exercise for newcomer. Go low on weight.

Barbell bridge (Pullover)

1. TAKE BRIDGE SPAN POSITION.

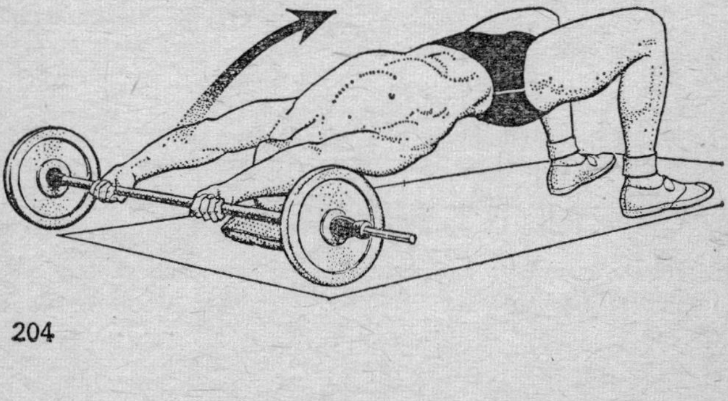

2. REACH ARMS BEHIND HEAD TO GRIP LOADED BARBELL PLACED BEHIND.
3. PULL OVER BAR AT ARMS' LENGTH TILL OVER CHEST (see CHEST).
4. LOWER AND REPEAT UNTIL NECK TIRED.

Note: bentarm pullover also OK (see CHEST). Inhale on lowering weight; exhale as YOU pullover. *Tough* exerciser.

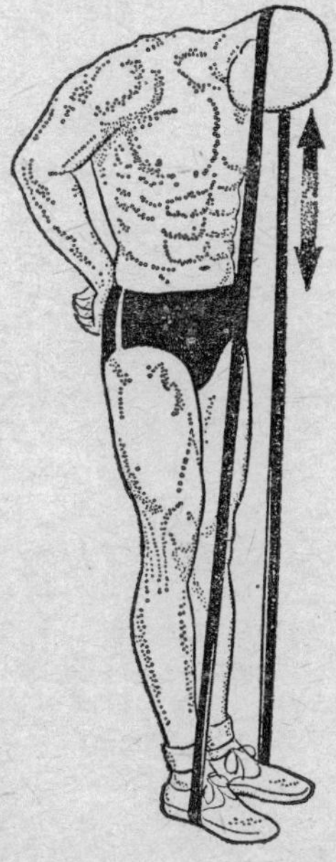

Inner tube puller
Stand on old cycle inner tube 2-footed and pass it round neck. Bob head up/down. 10 reps in 3 sets.

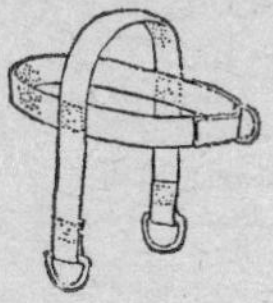

Head strapper
Make headstrap (as shown) from webbing (sewing-machine-

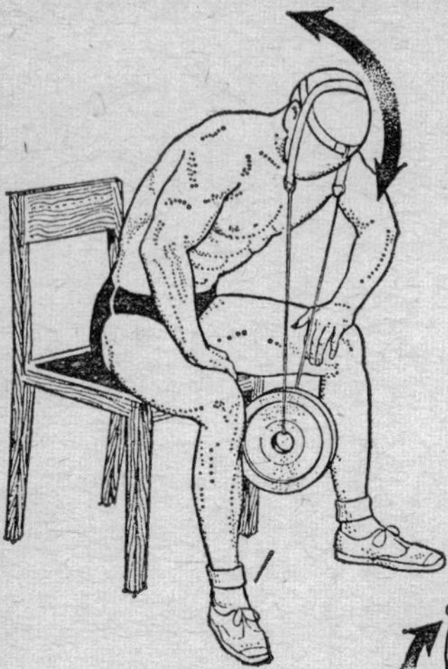

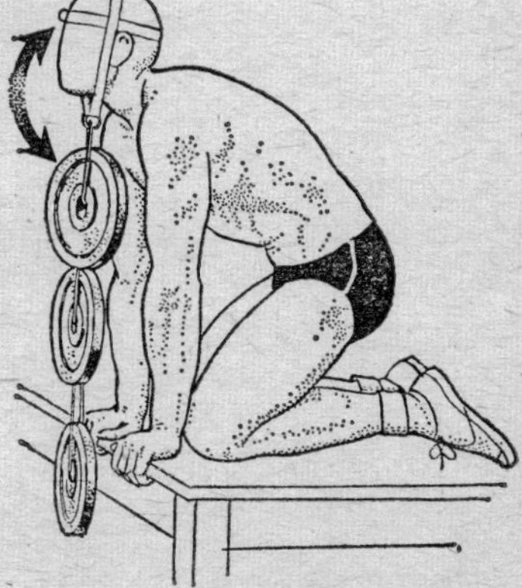

stitched). Pick old iron/scrap iron/etc., weight that = YOU doing 2–3 sets of 10–15 reps kneeling on chair/table and nodding head up/down.

Manual resistance

Mate clasps you round brow with hands or towel. YOU strain forward with head *steadily* aiming for head strapper-type reps until neck tired. Partner must NOT apply sudden pressure.

Also use his resistance for backward/sideways pull on neck muscles. 2–3 sets.

HEAD

HEAD : 9

YOUR HEAD is a Stone Age bone cage round the animal YOU. Every grimace/sneer/snarl shows the primitive beast in just one baring of your teeth (THE cardinal biological weapon of the human race with which to rive, rip, rend).

Extra to 10,000 teeth grindings and 5 million chews YOU do a year, can come the growl of the Caveman from lung air rushing over violin string thin vocal cords—a throwback to cavern shrieks/glacier groans/ape yells.

Do YOU bite at 50 lbs. pressure like a softy? Or exert that 200 lbs. champ of square-jawed MR TOUGH? Are YOUR eyes going, your voice gone? Bring back the Neolithic touch to your head. And become a force to be reckoned with.

WHAT YOUR HEAD WILL DO NOW

Make YOU more effective if you have never swum/fought/balanced before.

Defend YOUR life

When coat lapels grabbed in punchup be ready for assailant's head butting *you* in the face. Lower YOUR head so its boneplate of brow faces your opponent. Get in first by butting your forehead forward fast so its boneslab crashes on your antagonist's bridge of nose. HARD.

See better in the dark
Cut out torchlight which blinds night vision when you have a long way to go. Get eyes used to gloom by standing still for 5 minutes. Pupils will open wide scavenging for stray light rays. Other senses become more acute. Go slowly. Never trust eyes totally in limited light. If in doubt shine torch/match/lighter. Stop again after light goes out before moving on. Heed any sixth sense that danger lies ahead. Move cat-slow.

Nod goals
MR TOUGH heads good goals on beach or soccer field. With style. With brow-front. And neck muscles to flick ball with. And leg muscles to leap higher than the ball. And with arms/torso to help head propulsion. NEVER draw head in tortoise-fashion. Watch ball all the way. GO for it. HARD. Note: try softish ball at first.

See underwater
MR TOUGH is not afraid of water. Get head underwater. Grab shallow end rail if hesitant. Don't hold nose. Nor close eyes. Aim eyeballs/aim eyeballs/aim eyeballs at bath floor. Don't resurface to wipe eyes/face. Keep head down. Pick up objects thrown previously on to bath bottom. Scramble between mate's legs underwater. Aim eyeballs.

Make diving easy
THINK of head as counterweight which = vital aid to diving into water. Crouch half in water on shallow end steps, toes curled over a step, arms out, palms down. And HEAD DOWN. Pushoff with legs/feet/toes. And knife water *chin-on-chest.* Try diving next from: (1) sitting on bath edge; (2) squatting from same place; (3) standing crouched. Each time head DOWN. Note: head-raised dive = bad/flat water entry. Reason: you are sub-conciously afraid head-down approach will drive you through bath bottom. So you raise it at last second. Keep HEAD DOWN.

ALWAYS make yourself heard
Yell HELP! with most chance of being heard. Or ROAR at an attacker as YOU fight back for your life (a proved defence aid). Take deep breath. *Shout as loud as possible in your lowest register.* Keep foghorning—like Big Bertha bull horn which saves lost hunters in USA forests. Low-register roar better than shrill cries/screams/whistles.

Carry loads easily
Swing bucket of cement or similar on to skulltop with one arm (wear a cap or pad head). Balance it there one handed. Walk/

trot/climb ladder: keeping back straight, power coming from legs.
(*See also BACK.*)*

**= broad cloth band tied to top of packframe then passed round brow will lighten 100 lb. load, say, tremendously (using neck muscles via skull).*

Impress others with NEW you
Always hold head UP (for better posture). Also always face it straight at people you meet/talk to/pass. Eyes non-shifting. Grin.

Buck yourself up
By standing on head. Balance on head stands through practice:. Forget about breaking neck (you won't). Headstands irrigate brain with blood. Do a few minutes a day. Start headstanding against a wall. Then do it away from wall. Press with hands on floor. Bend legs. Get back straight. Kick UP hard. Have training mate hold you upright at first. Headstands *can* also relax body/help concentration/aid weight loss. Do headstands for several minutes in bathroom whenever you feel tense IF in good physical condition (NEVER if you have heart trouble). Proper Yoga headstand is shown (but takes hard practice).
(See also BRAIN/MIND.)

Refresh yourself when dozy and motorway driving
Spit on hands. Stick head out of window. Windsting on eye-sockets = YOU are woken up until next turnoff/service point.

Defend your eyesight automatically
DON'T RUB when something gets in your eye. Pull top lid over bottom lid. Hold for seconds. Then blink. Blink. Blink. Blink. Blink. NEVER RUB. Tear ducts will well eyes with water to clean them out. Blow nose as extra aid. Keep blinking.

MAKE A HEAD START TO-DAY

(*See also BODY.*)

Nose
Keep clean.

Sniff water up one nostril at a time from hand-hollow or head-tilt in shower. Pass it through mouth. Do it in SLOW stages (*skip if sinus afflicted*). At headcold sign add little disinfectant to water.

Note: Yoga cure for catarrh. Force thumb against right nostril, breathe gently in through left until lungs full. Lift thumb off, press against left nostril and breathe out through right nostril. Breathe in again through right and out through left. Then in through left and out through right. And so on. Always breathing in by nostril through which you have just breathed out. FOR 2 mins a morning.

Ears

NEVER mess about with ear wax (barrier against insects). Can cause infection which kills. Just wash daily. And see Dr. re sudden deafness.

Voice

Low clear voice = A MAN'S.

Protect pleasant voice. Colds/catarrh/fogs/wind/frost/coarse rich food/oversmoking ruin it. Vocal cords spider web delicate. Keep mouth shut. Breathe through nose.

Aim for MANLY voice + NEW shape. Buy battery tape recorder. Listen to Joe Soap. And for growl/twang/blur. Or slur. Or voice-fade at end of sente . . . Or worst phrases. Or wordstoboganning-together.

Golden rule: ALWAYS stress consonants (pre-stressed concrete of speech).

Pack muscle INTO voice (as in lats/delts/traps) with special toner for Cinderella muscles.

1. PLACE FLAT TOOTHBRUSH HANDLE ACROSS TEETH NEAR LIPS.
2. BITE ON THAT PLASTIC.
3. READ ALOUD FROM BOOK AS YOU . . .
4. MOVE LIPS BUT FREEZE TEETH. AIM TO . . .
5. SPEAK AS CLEARLY AS IF OBSTACLE NOT THERE.

Do this 15 minutes a day.

For first time ever tongue + lips have to fight. Result = new depth/vibrancy/sound. Above all . . . BE sincere when opening mouth.

FIGHT: speaking too fast (sowordsrunintoeachother); stressing SOME words AND NOT others; missing . . e TH's as in . . e definite article; failing to pronounce every letter in testers like Peter-Piper-picked-a-peck-of-pickled-peppers.

Toothbrush gripper = conquest of these targets.

Eyes

Warn you of attack—IF protagonist's shoulders move up/down/right/left (signal coming punch/kick).

Wear glasses WHEN you have too (never miss). Obtain best

spectacles possible. Find frames to suit face (so you WANT to wear them).

Bathe gritty/sore/red eyes in good optical bath solution. Tone eye muscles minus glasses (with rests between).

(a) Gaze at small object without blinking by focussing on high point then low point. Do 3 reps. Shut eyes. Then focus on right point, then left in 3 reps. Shut eyes.

(b) Stare hard at point of nose for several seconds. Then at distant point for same.

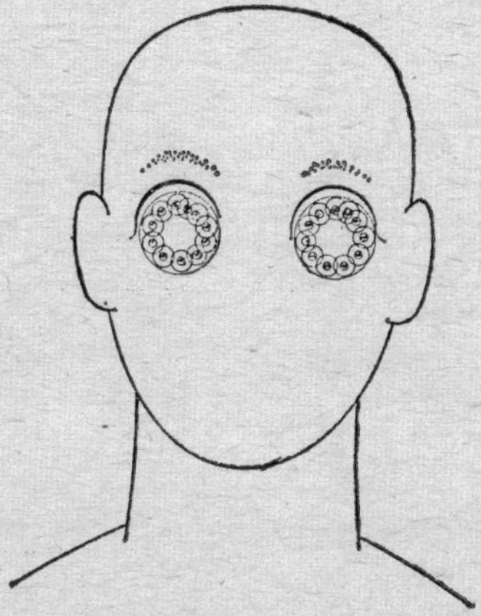

(c) Lock head straight to front. Use eyeball muscles to rol optical balls clockwise for 6 revolutions while gazing round outer limit (NOT moving head). See EVERYTHING.

(d) Repeat (c) rolling in anti-clockwise direction.

(e) Fix head still straight to front. Using eye muscle *only* flick gaze down from 12 o'clock to 6 o'clock pausing for 3 seconds at each time spot. Go clockwise round gaze-limit-circle thus: from 1 o'clock to 7 o'clock; 2 to 8; 3 to 9; 4 to 10; 5 to 11; 6 to 12; 7 to 5, etc. Memo: stay 3 seconds at each position.

(f) Repeat (e) anti-clockwise starting from 12 to 6; 11 to 5; 10 to 4; 9 to 3, etc.

Eyeball rolling = headstill vision fit for MR TOUGH.

Face

Revitalise YOUR 18 facial muscles.

IF going moonfaced *as chest gains space* (with power

programme) lose weight to lose muscleman jowls. And pull faces aplenty to keep skullfront youthful.

Grit teeth during hard resistance toners: powerful masseter muscles of jaws give strong chin contour.

Chew hard nosh (crusts/apples/carrots) well with primitive teeth grinding. Soft foods = neurotic trends in man (proven fact).

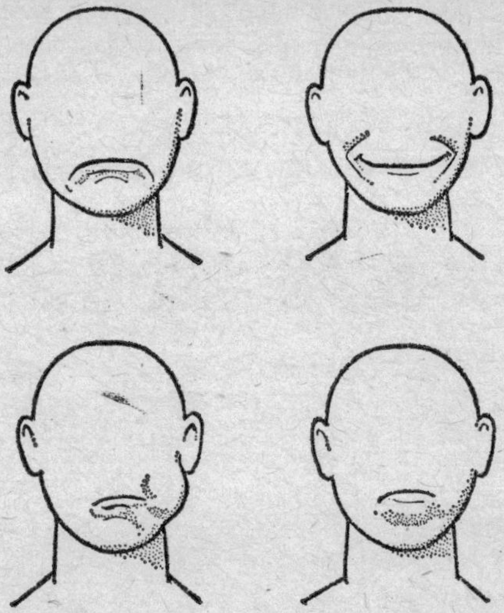

Yawn a lot (gaping mouth wide). Kill yourself laughing. Both stretch face.

Clamp teeth/lips together. Blow airball into lower lip zone. Hold 6 seconds balloon. Blow out. Bottle-up again. Inflate right cheek hard for 6 seconds. Release then pump-up top lip area. Give final 6 second airball dose to left cheek.

Drag back scalp muscles from hairline to smooth out brow wrinkles. Try for contractions rippling back from forehead to headrear. 6 second contractions.

Press teeth together. FORCE mouth corners down and out for 6 seconds. Then PULL up and out for 6.

BRAIN/MIND

BRAIN/MIND: 10

YOUR BRAIN is a rubbery moist haggis as big as a fist: 15 billion cells weighing as much as the Sunday joint are wrapped in a sheet of nerve fibres so wrinkled that pinned out flat it would cover a page of newspaper.

Fed by nerve impulses from 4 million pain flashpoints, 500,000 touch-triggers, 200,000 temperature indicators all over YOUR body, brain cells wave tentacle-fashion like surf-pounded seaweed (in pinkish-grey brain matter).

Are YOU swept by the tide? Or will YOU make YOUR own destiny? Your brain takes orders from YOU. Give yourself a Frankenstein shock to-day by electrifying YOUR brain into strongwilled action with immediate ACTION.

WHAT YOUR BRAIN WILL DO TO-DAY

Everything.

Always remember: it's ALL in the mind.

And WHAT a mind YOU have.: Nature's most powerful mechanism (yet when working at full pressure generating only one-25000th of a volt which wouldn't light a bike light. Moreover right side of brain controls left bodyside and viceversa. Note: as left side of brain usually strongest most of us = right handed + showing greater character on right face side. I.e. 2 photos, one made up from 2 left sides of YOUR face and other from 2 right sides will show 2 different people.

Use autosuggestion

Eat/sleep/drink POWer.* Cutout big photograph from muscle/sports/film magazine to show the male with THE toughnesses YOU desire. Paste photograph (to same scale) of YOUR head over his face. Aim to become that person in build YOURSELF (choose tall target if *you* are tall; short one if short yourself). Strive to grow into YOUR ideal. Stick snapshot of YOU on back of MR TOUGH'S title page. As YOU are NOW. Get to hate the smugness/fatness/unfitness you see. Determine to forge a NEW image from *to-day*. Write "S" or "M" or "P" or "MR. T" on bathroom mirror with soap. On cheque book/credit card/driving licence with feltpen. Carry big iron washer in pocket. Or sparkingplug/magnet/bolt as POWer memo.

*= KEEP muscle-aim to self so YOUR enthusiasm is always kettlehot—don't spout it away by shouting the odds.

Note: KNOW using brain as overdrive will = REAL results in 4 months; a Colossus-build (compared with what you are now) in 12 months; muscle-mag-photo-build in 36–120 months of HARD training.

Think SUBconsciously

Workout a problem's pros/cons on paper to smash that problem. List fors/againsts side by side. Puzzle it out. Chew it over. Rack YOUR brains. AND everyone else's (jot those opinions down too).

Leave off—*still* puzzling.

Make love. Smoke cigarettes. Drive car. Hoist weights. Go running. Sleep. Pedal cycle. Paddle canoe. Climb rocks. Relax on sand/snow/water. Shoot gun/bow/rapids. Drink beer. Watch football/TV/birds. Mow lawn. Wash motor bike. Clean typewriter. Play table tennis. Read paperback. And . . .

Answer WILL come. May not be inspiration-flash but be result of more figuring with pen to paper. Heed BRAIN'S decision (as opposed to HEART'S). Subconscious thinking = a clear answer.

MR TOUGH prefers to follow brain rather than heart.

Prove brighter than YOU think

NEVER underestimate YOUR own IQ, nor overestimate anyone else's. Prove brighter than YOU or friends think YOU are (just as your body is tougher than you thought). Kick lazybrains by getting excited over becoming MR TOUGH. Brain will respond. IF you have it in YOU to make a MR TOUGH (without dropping-out en route): you *have* excellent IQ (all successful bodybuilders have).

NOURISH YOUR BRAIN NOW

Think about it.

With exercise

PHYSICAL exercise boosts mental powers. Relieves mental

blocks/breakups/tensions. Makes YOU happy/chuffed/madeup. Mind AND body as close as your 1st/2nd fingers crossed. Exercise puts "muscle" in brain tissue. PHYSICAL workouts = untroubled mind/deep sleep/refreshed awakening. And keener reflexes.

With right attitude

Say: "I am growing tougher all the time." NEVER say: "I am MR TOUGH". That last thought *now* = a lie. And a mental dangerpoint. Always tell yourself the truth. NEVER believe what you most definitely are not.

With anxiety/tension/stress throwout

TENSION = throat/midriff/chest pain. Rashes and spots and boils. Alarming illnesses masquerades. For labourers *and* executives. ALL = brain/mind warning YOU are not living wisely.

1. NEVER TAKE ON MORE THAN YOU CAN HANDLE (THIS INC. YOUR MR TOUGH PROGRAMME: KEEP IT WELL IN LIMITS).
2. NEVER GO SHORT OF SLEEP.
3. KEEP EXERCISING THROUGHOUT LIFE.
4. PUT YOUR HOUSE IN ORDER WHEN HEART IS OVERULING BRAIN IN DAFT ACTIONS.

Know: prolonged tension cuts down lifespan.

With ACTion

When depressed/worried/distressed ACT physically to get brain moving. DO something (even wrong thing better than nothing). Helps you rationalize problem, beats fear. Get on train/in car/by foot *to* whatever is wrong. Face it. Sort it out. Brain will release hidden resources from you to face any crisis. IF you act physically first.

RELEASE THE GIANT INSIDE YOU

Everyone can do more than they ever dreamt possible. Let brain motivate YOU to becoming MR TOUGH.

Get ideas

Bombard brain with muscle ideas. From books/mags/life. Admire strength and POWer. Visit gymnasiums. Strongman exhibitions. Karate/judo/aikaido displays. Canoe slaloms. Sports fields. Highland Games. Meet strongmen from all over. Share ideas. Hammer YOUR brain with impressions of strength. Relate everything to terms of strength. And human endeavour.

Let ideas get YOU

Like idea of MR TOUGH. Of being square shouldered. Of

having muscle-roped arms. Of gaining iron fists. Of a tanned skin. Of hanging good clothes on polished limbs. Of sitting back easily behind wheel/on saddle/in cockpit. Of silent striding. Of hawkeyed scanning. Of sureness of movement of quietness of manner. Of wristwatch glanced at/lighter flicked/cheque written with unseen muscle flex. Of clean-limbed relaxing. Of luggage-grid-landed suitcase with wristflick. Of always knowing YOU are up to it.

Become enthusiastic
NOTHING kicks brain into action like excitement. Grow it over becoming MR TOUGH. See YOURSELF as anything but MR SOFT one day. Soak YOURSELF in secret self-improvement plan. DARE yourself to begin to-day.

Dare yourself
Becoming MR TOUGH is ambition. Any ambitious venture needs courage. Again—*dare* YOURSELF to start.

Get on with it
NOW.

Act physically and brain will lead YOU through right on to MR TOUGH target. Whenever progress seems at a standstill: keep going. Batter each obstacle en route. Never give up. You will pass through each challenge (*like athlete getting second wind after stitch*).

USE BRAIN STAMINA TO FUEL YOUR GIANT

By planning on paper.

Plan in stages
NEVER see MR TOUGH objective as a WHOLE. Breakdown aim into phases that will not dishearten. Makeup YOUR own easy stages of muscle construction. Follow this: bulldozing *each* section in turn then moving on to next. Until YOU are MR TOUGH.

Act as an individual
Work out YOUR easy stages YOURSELF (see BODY). No 2 MR SOFTS ever reached strength the same way. Consider your build/age/condition. And aim for a set standard personal to YOU. Never follow blindly as in a tunnel any one set of exercises—but experiment. Variants CAN be made from basic battle plan. Such a foundation for Oxfam Ad type (first 6–8 weeks) is . . .

Warm up by "cleaning" barbell.

1. Press from neckback. 4 sets of 6 reps.
2. Breathing squat. 4 sets of 8.
3. Bench press with barbell. 4 sets of 6.

4. Barbell rowing. 3 sets of 8.
5. Deadlift. 4 sets of 5.

Thus skinny man is NOT burningup vital energy to exhaust him. Whereas he could be shattered by routine foundation for heavier man which might be . . .

Warm up by "cleaning" barbell.

1. Press from neckback. 3 sets of 8 reps.
2. Seated single arm curl. 3 sets of 8.
3. Upright rowing. 3 sets of 10.
4. Breathing squat. 3 sets of 12.
5. Pullover with dumbells. 3 sets of 10.
6. Bench press with barbell. 3 sets of 10.
7. Single arm rowing. 3 sets of 12 an arm.
8. Standing heel raise. 4 sets of 15.
9. Sidebend with dumbell. 2 sets of 30 a side.

Use BRAIN to determine how *heavy* weights should *be* (see BODY). Use BRAIN to check YOU really do struggle on last 2 reps of a set. Use BRAIN to know you *are* gaining POWer (and NEED to add extra weight as resistance around every 4th workout). Use BRAIN to *keep* you working HARD (but not to flakeout point).

And advance as far as YOU want

To MR FIT/MR TOUGH/MR SUPERTOUGH. And to ANY stage inbetween. To whatever stage YOU are happy at. YOUR brain/mind/inclination decides progress speed (whether cart horse slow or runaway mustang style). Keep STICKING at it. AND when you reach fitness happiness level for YOU: work HARD to stay there. NEVER slip/slide/skid back to the dreaded MR SOFT. Keep BRAIN alert to ALL possibilities of extending your strength. NEVER just plod on using same old exercise routines month after month. Feed the mind with POWer ideas. ACT on best of them.

Creating MR SUPERTOUGH

ADVANCED POWer training = Nuclear War on MUSCLES. Can only be declared (IF you want to win) 6–12 months after start of regular weight training warfare. IF *you* want it enough. IF *you* are showing advancing results. IF *you* throw ALL *mental* resources into it. Advanced POWer Game = systems like:

CHEATING: with mammoth weights.* And doing exercises in strictly non-strict style. Bonus = YOU smash sticking barriers; pack extra bulk/POWer; make weights you go back to using in strict-style seem hydrogen-filled. THUS: barbell curl cheating style = body heave with little backbend (not TOO much) to bring bar to chest; cheat bench press = usual start with arms propping bar above chest BUT shoving bar back after it nudges chest with bodyarch at each rep so glutes lift off bench in mini-bridge position; cheat bentover rowing = faster-than-usual lug from floor with chest coming down to meet bar on its way up so making 2 movements in 1; cheat upright towing motion = bar at hang held with narrow grasp is lowered down thighs as body bends forward from waist and is then hauled back up to chin with *some* backbend; cheat standing triceps stretch = start at full arms stretch overhead followed by lowering weight to neckback while bending knees slightly and THEN straightening arms to press load back up while simultaneously snapping legs straight; cheating lateral raise = bringing dumbells from hang up and sideways by bending torso slightly forward and suddenly straightening up.

*= Yes, mammoth weights *compared* with those you have used so far in ordinary strict-style weight training. E.g.: cheat bench press allows YOU to tote 20/30 lbs. more iron; cheat upright rowing allows 10/15 lbs. more; cheat lateral raise allows 5/10 lbs. more. Approx.

Note: CHEATING methods are never used continuously/ALL at once/by beginners. Best used to boost backward body parts lacking bulk for 6–8 week session. Only 1/2 exercises in whole programme should be cheated-on. And then with *combo* of strict exercise for that body part too. E.g.: for BICEPS do cheating curl with barbell followed by lighter dumbell curl in strict style. Return to strict style AFTER 6–8 weeks cheater spell (and weights floatup).

More SUPERTOUGH treatment

Enough?

Or does BRAIN crave/want/order more? BRAIN motivation backedup by GROWING body needs more and more advanced strength system to feed on. Like.

FLUSHING: by pumping blood into muscle until fibres are gorged up to 1 in. bigger after workout (deflation time: about 30 mins.). Arm flushing, say = bicep after bicep exercise, set after set until muscle ready to burst. YOU pick muscle group and bombard it with 9 consecutive sets made up of 3 different exercises (each hitting from NEW angle). E.g.: for ARMS never choose 3 light movements BUT ensure one is heavy poundage exercise. Thus: do single dumbell concentration curls, yes; but followup with hefty 2-handed barbell curls to add meat to pumpedup feeling. And DO use loaf ALL time (even to order of choosing body parts to flush). Don't skip from one end of body to other. Move blood to adjacent areas so gorge-flow has least ways to travel. E.g.: flush chest/arms/delts in order like chain links.

SUPER SETS: where exercises alternate in FAST succession

spilling out POWer/bulk and shape/pump. Biceps then triceps, biceps then triceps, biceps then triceps. I.e.: YOU do 3 sets of 2 exercises *alternating a set of one with a set of the other*. Super sets work for opposing sectors of same muscle group. Biceps/triceps, say. Often a chunky barbell movement followed by a lighter dumbell one. E.g.: CHEST could = bench press *then* flying exercise.

SPLIT SYSTEM: is for control so runaway muscles will NOT trip. So they can recuperate after HEAVY thrashing. DO torso MON, legs TUES, layoff WED, torso THURS, legs FRI, layoff SAT/SUN. Then repeat for rest of 6–8 week session. Benefits = more pinpoint concentration possible; more rugged muscle flogging possible (you forget legs on torso day); more sets and extra exercises possible for each body half. Can take briefer time too for busy man.

TRI-BOMBING: means machine gunning same body part from 3 different trajectories (very advanced). Select 1 exercise for bulk, 1 for shape, 1 for muscle definition. And only when super sets fail to bring on a laggard body zone. E.g.: DELTS = bench press for bulk; dips for fullness plus impressive delts/pects tieup; bench press with dumbells for pecs definition. NEVER use tri-bombing for vanity so ONE body gets out of balance with REST of YOU. NO more than 2 body parts should be tri-bombed in a session. 10 per cent less weight than normal is used. And each set of the 3 separate exercises makes ONE tri-bomb set. Keep knocking them out, MR SUPERTOUGH, until *you* feel on fire.

QUALITY TRAINING: is fast/fast/minipause schedule done flatout (BUT never skimped). YOU rest as little as possible done flatout (BUT never skimped). YOU rest as little as possible inbetween reps/sets. Not for colossal bulk/POWer *but* for muscle definition/shape. Choose 3 exercises for each bodypart to blitz from ALL angles (and do, approx., 5–6 sets for 6–8 reps using heftiest weights YOU can tote in GOOD style). Pick exercises which pinpoint specific muscle NOT which blanket whole muscle slab with rocketfire. Hit each muscle HARD/FAST/DEADON. E.g.: use wide grip chins (for back) instead of bentover rowing; concentration curls instead of barbell cheating curl; etc. Never sacrifice strict style here for SPEED.

DIG for Victory

Dig/dig/dig deep into scientific bodybuilding books/mags/talk. Make mates from best gyms where strongmen meet. Inspire BRAIN to guide YOU to heights for stature YOU have in mind. Strive to cruise through POWer plan at right happiness level (YOU are in wrong stratosphere if tense/edgy/prickly through POWer aim). MR SUPERTOUGH goes for even more punishment once he is happy (he may often have had to back off the throttle from time to time en route) . . . with GIANT SETS/POWER STOPS/BURNS. Even SPLITTING THE SPLIT SYSTEM.

HARNESS YOUR GIANT FOR EVERYTHING

NOT just in PHYSICAL things. In EVERYthing. In Life. Carry out same principles in work/play/living as YOU do to grow MUSCLE. BOMBard your brain with new ideas. Work on THE ideas which *get you* with enthusiasm/zest/keenness. Give them ALL. They are the bonuses of LIFE. Work hard on these ideas. Expand them. Act on them. Dig into them. Get excited/thrilled/deadkeen. Let BRAIN shoot you through (and also flash redlight warnings). Change job/recreation/life to the ONE you want above all else: to the one YOU are/will be good at. Get out of tradition/custom/habit (yes, RUT) to rocket into a full life. YOU don't have to go to university to get broader outlook than many graduates. MR TOUGH is graduate of *life*. Whenever you can moan—go like a bomb to get to nomoan level. E.g.: YOU hate YOUR job. Change to whatever YOU want to do and start from scratch. Give it everything. As YOU battle YOU will unleash resources of MIND/BRAIN/BODY that you never knew existed outside Supermen. Just believe in YOURSELF (above all else). IF you fail, grope back up and start again learning from mistakes. BUT quest for ideas initially often best guarantee YOU *will* succeed. Sensory bombardment (from people/places/books) = golden ideas which GET you. YOU never know what is "YOU" until you try. Exercising physically for MR TOUGH activates YOUR brain and helps from word GO! So ideas flow until YOU say: "That's ME!" From then on: aim to succeed in that field. Get to know its leaders. Read ALL you can on it. Collect colleagues good at it. And DARE yourself to GROW.

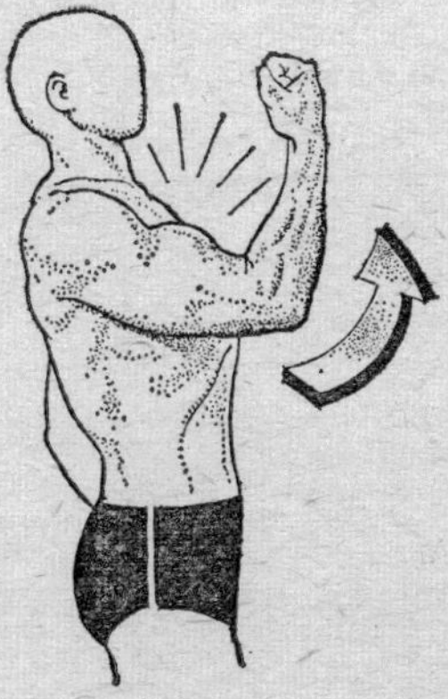